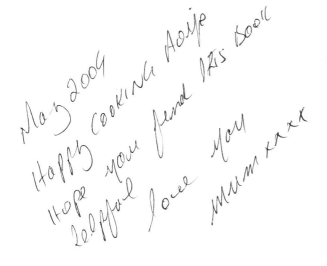

May 2009
Happy cooking Aoife
Hope you find this book
helpful. love you
mum xxxx

Irresistibles for the Irritable

by Sue Shepherd

Photography by Martin Shepherd

Gluten Free

Wheat Free

Coeliac Disease

Lactose Intolerance

Fructose Malabsorption

Irritable Bowel Syndrome

Acknowledgments
This book has become a reality because of the support and encouragement of so many. Thanks to my husband, Martin, a wonderful designer, photographer and friend. And for my Pop: a great supporter, sadly missed. Sincere thanks also to my lovely family and friends, to work colleagues, and to past patients. Your support and enthusiasm has made the adventure of producing book number two a great one.

As I have coeliac disease, I know the limitations and frustrations that a special diet can bring. However, I also know how much I enjoy the foods I eat! Great tasting food is a right, not a luxury. So, for all my past patients with coeliac disease, irritable bowel syndrome, fructose malabsorption, lactose intolerance – this is a book written for you. For my future patients, and for those with these conditions whom I may never meet, I have written it for you, too. I want you to thoroughly enjoy these great tasting, friendly recipes.

Author
Sue Shepherd
B. App. Sci. (Health Promotion), M. Nutrition & Dietetics, A.P.D.

Design and Photography
Martin Shepherd

Publisher
First published in Australia in 2004
By Shepherd Works Pty Ltd
PO Box 6015 Croydon North, Victoria 3136, Australia
ABN 53 095 268 170
www.coeliac.com.au
Printed in China

©2004 Shepherd Works Pty Ltd
PO Box 6015 Croydon North, Victoria 3136, Australia

National Library of Australia Cataloguing-in-Publication data:
Shepherd, Sue.
Irresistibles for the Irritable.
Includes index.
ISBN – 0-9751957-0-0
1.Gluten-free diet – Recipes 2. Celiac Disease - Diet therapy - Recipes. I. Shepherd, Martin.
II. Title.

641.563

contents

Coeliac Disease

Irresistibles for the Irritable contains a delicious range of gluten free recipes. A gluten free diet is required for the management of coeliac disease.

Coeliac disease is a medically diagnosed condition of an intolerance to gluten in the diet. Gluten is the protein component of wheat, rye, barley and possibly oats. In people with coeliac disease, gluten causes damage to the lining of the small intestine (villi). As a result, the ability to absorb nutrients is dramatically decreased and people can become very unwell. Typical symptoms can include bloating, wind, pain, diarrhoea or constipation (or a combination of both), fatigue and iron deficiency.

Coeliac disease is a lifelong condition treated by a diet free from all gluten. This prevents further damage to the villi and allows them to return to normal, so that nutrients can be properly absorbed.

The gluten free diet permits fruits, vegetables, plain meat, fish and chicken, legumes and lentils, most dairy foods, oils, butter and margarines.

Breads, pasta and cereals can be made from alternative sources, including corn, rice, soy, potato and tapioca to name a few. There are many specialty gluten free products available.

For most people diagnosed as requiring a gluten free diet, the change in lifestyle is often overwhelming. Learning which foods are suitable, and which foods are no longer permitted in the diet is time consuming at first, and the diet can seem very restrictive. *Irresistibles for the Irritable* allows you to fully enjoy the great tastes of a gluten free diet.

Every effort has been made to indicate the gluten free ingredients used in *Irresistibles for the Irritable* (see p. 132 for more information). However, it is essential to read the ingredients list on the packaging of all food products you buy, to ensure they are gluten free. The recipes in this book comply with the Australian gluten free food standard at the time of printing. The author does not accept any responsibility for changes to the gluten free status of foods after the time of printing, nor for differences in gluten free standards in other countries.

Lactose Intolerance

Lactose intolerance can be a cause of symptoms of irritable bowel syndrome. Additionally, many people with coeliac disease can have a secondary lactose intolerance. In such people, the lactose intolerance is usually only temporary, caused by the gluten-damage in the small intestine. In others, however, it is a condition that will remain for life.

Lactose is a naturally occurring sugar that is found in cow, goat and sheep milk. Typically, in people with lactose intolerance, the body stops making enough of the enzyme lactase, which breaks down the sugar lactose. However, people can differ in the severity of their intolerance. Most people are able to tolerate small amounts of lactose in their diet.

Lactose is present in large amounts in milk, ice cream and custard. It is present in moderate amounts in yoghurt and soft/unripened cheeses (e.g. cottage, ricotta, quark, cream cheeses). Cream contains a minimal amount of lactose. Hard/ripened cheeses (cheddar, tasty, parmesan, camembert, edam, gouda, blue vein, mozzarella, etc.) and butter are virtually free of lactose.

The majority of recipes in *Irresistibles for the Irritable* are lactose free or contain only minimal amounts of lactose. Recipes that require modification (if the amount of lactose in the serve is high) are marked with a symbol •. See the recipe hints section on page 132 for more information.

Fructose Malabsorption

Fructose malabsorption is a condition where the small intestine is impaired in its ability to absorb fructose (a naturally occurring sugar). Fructose malabsorption is a different condition to hereditary fructose intolerance.

When fructose is not absorbed properly in the small intestine, it can travel through to the large intestine where bacterial fermentation can cause symptoms of irritable bowel syndrome. These include bloating, wind, pain, nausea, diarrhoea and/or constipation.

Although fructose is present in one form or another in virtually every fruit, and in many vegetables and grains, not every food source of fructose needs to be avoided by people with fructose malabsorption.

The most commonly consumed problem foods are:
Fruits: Apple, pear, mango, watermelon, quince, paw paw, lychee, guava and persimmon. In excess, the following are problematic: dried fruit, fruit juice, tomato paste.
Vegetables: onion, spring onion, leek, asparagus, artichoke, Jerusalem artichoke, witlof, chicory, radicchio, dandelion greens.
Others: honey, coconut cream and large quantities of wheat. Fructose, fruit juice sweeteners (apple juice concentrate, pear pastes) and high fructose corn syrups are ingredients that are increasing in their use by the food industry. They are concentrated in fructose and are a problem in large amounts.

You will note some ingredients will be specified to be "gluten free". Gluten is in wheat, rye, barley and possibly oats. People with fructose malabsorption find wheat is a problem food when consumed in large amounts; however, they can eat rye, barley and oats. Although "gluten free" is not specifically required for people with fructose malabsorption, as every recipe in this cookbook is gluten free, they are all also wheat free.

All the recipes in *Irresistibles for the Irritable* are formulated without the above-mentioned problem ingredients. (If onions are used, they are discarded and not present in the final form of the dish). This is the first cookbook to cater for fructose malabsorption.

Although the recipes are all formulated with ingredients that are suitable for fructose malabsorption, if you suffer from this condition, ensure that you limit your serving size of any fruit- or tomato-based dish to that which is indicated on the recipe. Consuming large quantities of even "safe" fruits can cause symptoms.

If you have noticed you feel better on a wheat-free diet, you may have fructose malabsorption. However, coeliac disease may also be a possibility. You should discuss tests for coeliac disease with your doctor (see next section on irritable bowel syndrome for more information). It is possible to have both coeliac disease and fructose malabsorption.

Irritable Bowel Syndrome

Irritable bowel syndrome (IBS) is a condition that affects approximately 15% of the population. Symptoms can include abdominal pain or discomfort, and change in bowel habits (diarrhoea, constipation or a combination of both). Wind, bloating, and nausea are also common. These symptoms can fluctuate in their severity from day to day and week to week.

The diagnosis is made on the pattern of symptoms. One condition that can mimic IBS is coeliac disease. Simple screening blood tests are now readily available. Ask your doctor for blood tests to investigate for coeliac disease. You do need to be eating gluten in the diet for the tests to be useful. If the tests are positive, it does not absolutely confirm coeliac disease. A small bowel biopsy is still considered the gold standard for diagnosis. Talk to your doctor or gastroenterologist for more information about coeliac disease.

There is no one diet that will suit every person who suffers from IBS. There may be many food triggers. People with IBS often find a reduced wheat and reduced dairy diet are helpful in minimising symptoms. Could it be that you may suffer from fructose malabsorption (wheat) or lactose intolerance (dairy)? It may be worth your while to trial a reduced intake of these problematic foods to see if your symptoms improve. As all recipes in *Irresistibles for the Irritable* are wheat free, and most are lactose free, it is likely they will be suitable for you.

High-fat foods often aggravate symptoms of IBS. Therefore, low-fat ingredients are encouraged. In many instances, these are specified in the ingredients listing. Most recipes in *Irresistibles for the Irritable* are not high in fat.

Sorbitol is a component in many stone fruits, and may also cause symptoms of IBS in sensitive people. Some recipes in *Irresistibles for the Irritable* use stone fruits. However, alternatives are suggested when indicated with •. See the recipe hints section on page 132.

For more information: www.coeliac.com.au

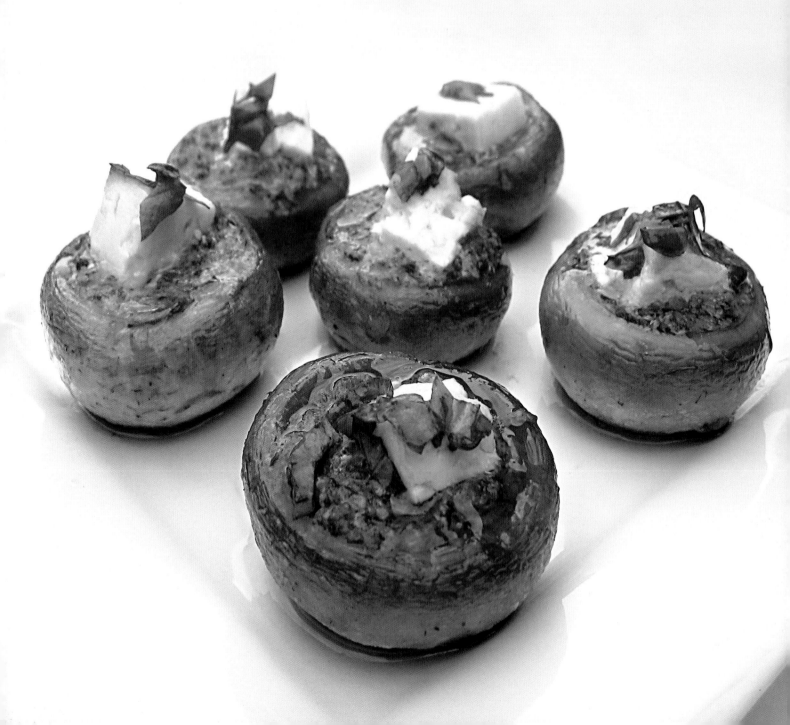

starters

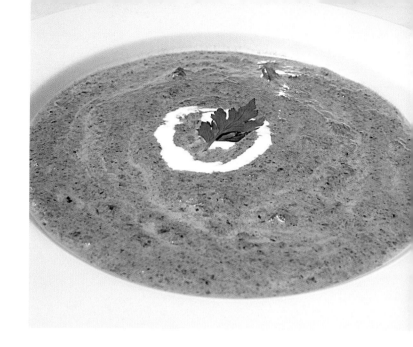

CHICKEN NOODLE SOUP

8 cups (2L) gluten free chicken stock
3 tsp fresh ginger, grated
4 kaffir lime leaves
500g chicken breast fillets, cut into very thin slices
200g dried rice noodle squares (5cm)
3 bunches (330g) baby bok choy, rinsed, separated
1/2 cup (25g) fresh bean sprouts
2 tsp gluten free soy sauce

In a large heavy-based saucepan, bring chicken stock, ginger, and kaffir lime leaves to the boil. Add raw chicken slices, and reduce heat. Cook, simmering for 5 minutes. Add rice noodles, bok choy leaves and bean sprouts. Continue to simmer over low heat for 5 minutes, until rice noodles tender. Remove lime leaves. Stir through soy sauce and serve.

Hint: Rice noodle squares are available from Asian grocers. Regular dried rice noodles can also be used.

Serves 4

MUSHROOM SOUP

3 Tbsp butter
1kg mushrooms, sliced
3 Tbsp gluten free cornflour
6 cups (1500ml) gluten free beef stock
2/3 cup (165ml) white wine
2 tsp ground mustard powder
1 1/3 cups (340ml) reduced fat cream
4 Tbsp fresh parsley, chopped
salt, freshly ground black pepper to taste

In a large heavy-based saucepan over medium heat, melt butter and sauté sliced mushrooms. Stir constantly until mushrooms soften and slightly brown. Mix cornflour with a little beef stock to form a paste. Add remaining beef stock slowly to cornflour paste, mixing well to ensure smooth consistency. Pour over mushrooms, and add white wine and mustard. Cook over medium heat, uncovered, for 15 minutes, stirring occasionally. Remove from heat and stir through cream. Purée with hand-held blender. Return to heat, until almost boiling. Stir through parsley and season with salt and pepper.

Hint: If lactose intolerant, this recipe is unsuitable.

Serves 4

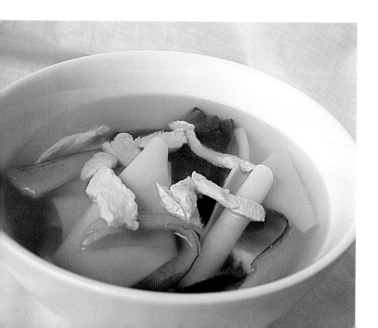

LETTUCE CUPS

2 Tbsp sesame oil
2 cloves garlic, crushed
2 tsp fresh ginger, finely grated
500g pork mince
190g can champignons, drained, sliced
290g can water chestnuts, finely chopped
1/3 cup (45g) bamboo shoots, finely chopped
1 Tbsp fresh coriander, chopped
2 Tbsp lemon juice
1 1/2 Tbsp gluten free sweet chilli sauce
1 tsp fish sauce
6 small-medium iceberg lettuce leaves, rinsed

In a medium frying pan, heat oil and sauté garlic and ginger, until browned. Add pork mince, and stir-fry over high heat for 3 to 4 minutes or until pork cooked. Break up any mince lumps. Add champignons, water chestnuts, bamboo shoots, coriander, lemon juice, chilli and fish sauces. Continue to stir-fry for a further 2 minutes. Spoon mixture onto lettuce leaves. Serve immediately.

Serves 6

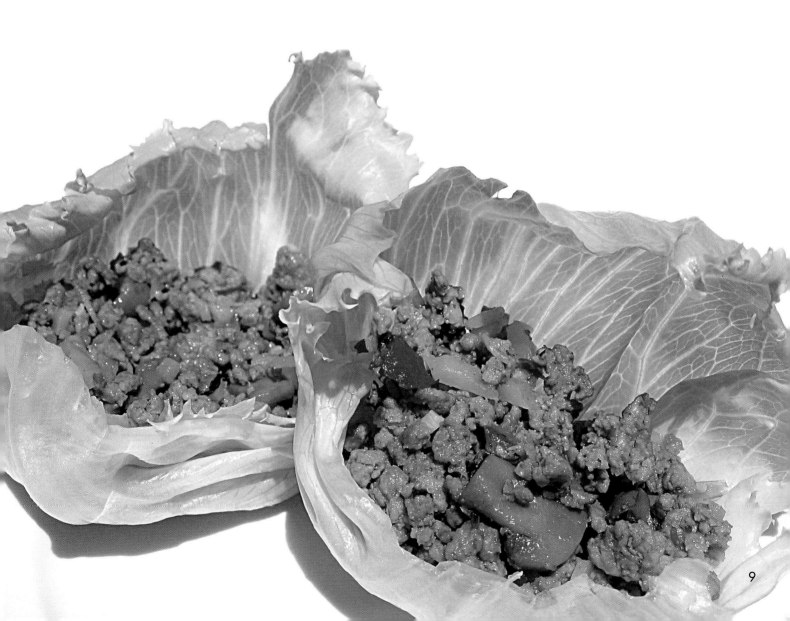

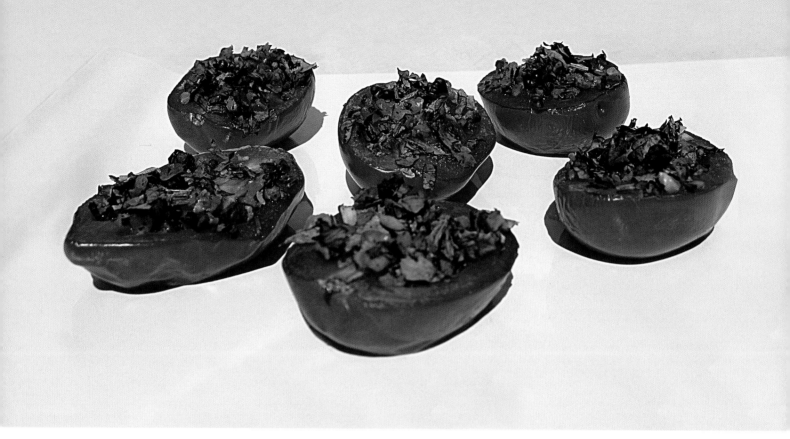

TASTY TOMATO BITES WITH PINE NUT TOPPING

1/3 cup (60g) pine nuts, finely chopped
1 1/2 Tbsp lemon rind, finely grated
1/2 clove garlic, crushed
1/3 cup fresh parsley, finely chopped
8 small (520g) Roma tomatoes, halved
2 Tbsp balsamic vinegar

Pre-heat oven to 180°C. Combine pine nuts, lemon rind, garlic and parsley in a bowl.
Place tomatoes, cut side up, on baking tray. Drizzle tomatoes with balsamic vinegar, then
top with prepared topping. Bake in pre-heated oven for 15 to 20 minutes, or until tomatoes
softened. Serve warm.

Serves 16

ASIAN NOODLE CAKES WITH CHILLI SAUCE

375g dried flat rice noodles (5mm wide)
1/3 cup fresh coriander, chopped
3 cloves garlic, crushed
2 tsp fresh ginger, grated
1/2 tsp Chinese five spice
3 eggs, lightly whisked
2 Tbsp sesame oil
1/3 cup (85ml) gluten free sweet chilli sauce
2 Tbsp gluten free cornflour
salt to taste
cooking spray

Chilli sauce
1/2 cup (125ml) gluten free sweet chilli sauce, extra
1 Tbsp plum jam
1/2 tsp gluten free soy sauce

Fill a large bowl with hot water. Roughly break up rice noodles into 5 to 10cm pieces. Soak for 4 to 5 minutes or until tender, then drain and rinse under cool water.

Transfer to a large bowl and add coriander, garlic, ginger, five-spice powder, eggs, sesame oil, chilli sauce, cornflour and salt. Mix until well combined.

Heat a large heavy-based frying pan over medium heat. Spray pan and inside of egg rings with cooking spray. Position greased egg rings in pan and place spoonfuls of the noodle mixture to fill the egg rings. Ensure noodle mixture is well packed into egg rings, but not overflowing. Cook for 2 to 3 minutes each side or until golden brown. Remove from pan and run a knife around the inside of each ring to remove noodle cakes. Set cooked noodle cakes aside on a plate, covered, to keep warm. Repeat with the remaining mixture. Serve warm with prepared sauce.

Chilli sauce: Combine sweet chilli sauce, plum jam and soy sauce in a small mixing bowl. Stir until well combined.

Makes 16

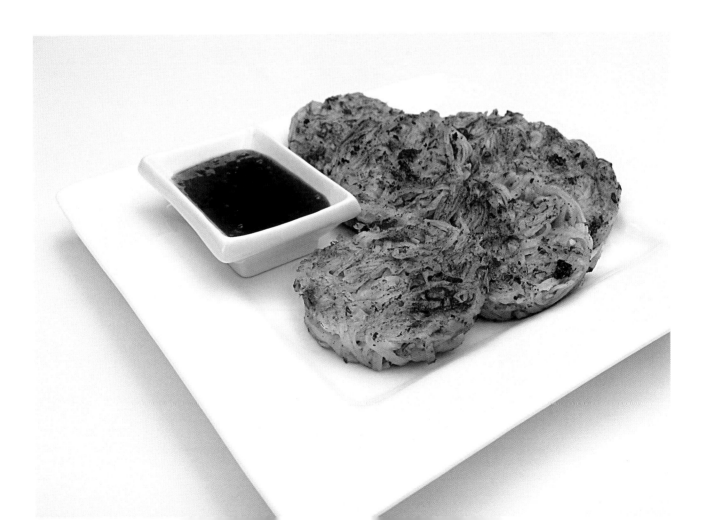

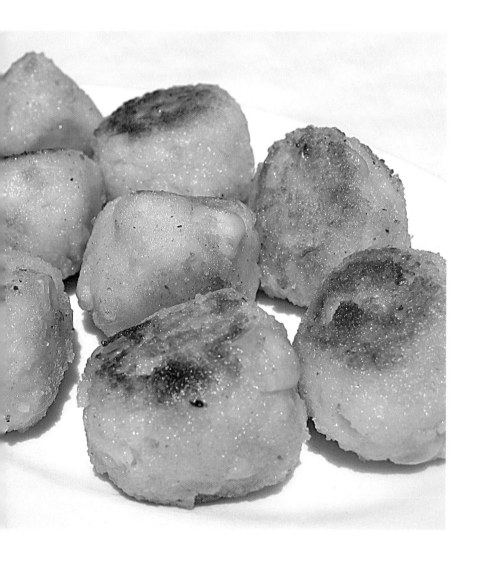

CHEESE AND CORN BALLS

3/4 cup (160g) long grain rice
3 cups (750ml) strong gluten free chicken stock
3/4 cup (90g) parmesan cheese, grated
3/4 cup (150g) corn kernels
1 egg, beaten
1/3 cup (40g) gluten free breadcrumbs
1 cup (120g) gluten free breadcrumbs, extra, to coat
canola oil

Heat chicken stock in a large saucepan and cook rice until tender. Drain any excess liquid, and let stand for 2 minutes. Transfer to a medium mixing bowl and stir in cheese and corn kernels. Set aside and allow to cool.

Pre-heat oven to 150°C. When rice mixture has cooled to room temperature, mix in beaten egg and breadcrumbs. Mixture should now be firm enough to roll into golf ball-size balls. Add more breadcrumbs if required. Pour extra gluten free breadcrumbs into a shallow bowl.
Toss formed rice balls in breadcrumbs until well coated. Heat a little canola oil in a frying pan over medium-high heat. When pan is warmed, add rice balls to frying pan, cooking in batches of ten at a time. Toss regularly; cook until evenly browned all over. Set aside on a baking tray and keep warm in the pre-heated oven. Add more oil to warm frying pan and repeat the process until all the balls are cooked.
Serve warm.

Makes 30

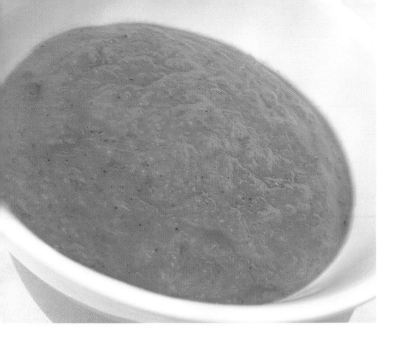

ROASTED PUMPKIN AND CHESTNUT SOUP

2kg pumpkin, peeled, cut into 2cm pieces
2 Tbsp olive oil
2 cups (500g) chestnut purée
8 cups (2L) strong gluten free vegetable stock
2 tsp ground ginger
1 cup (250ml) reduced fat milk *
salt, freshly ground black pepper to taste

Pre-heat oven to 180°C. Place pumpkin pieces on baking tray and drizzle with olive oil. Bake in pre-heated oven, turning occasionally, for 30 to 40 minutes or until cooked and browned.

Add puréed chestnuts, cooked pumpkin, vegetable stock and ground ginger to large stockpot. Simmer over medium-low heat, uncovered for 15 to 20 minutes, stirring occasionally. Remove from heat, add milk and purée with hand held blender until even in texture. Taste, season with salt and pepper.

Hint: Chestnut purée is available from gourmet delis. It is worth the effort to find.

Serves 4   * See recipe hints p.132

CURRIED POTATO AND PARSNIP SOUP

2 medium (350g) parsnips, peeled, cut into 2cm pieces
4 medium (720g) potatoes, peeled, cut into 2cm pieces
1 Tbsp canola oil
6 cups (1500ml) gluten free vegetable stock
1 tsp gluten free curry powder (more according to taste)
1 cup (250ml) reduced fat evaporated milk *

In a large heavy-based saucepan, heat oil over medium heat. Add parsnip and potato pieces and sauté for 3 to 5 minutes, stirring regularly until lightly browned. Add vegetable stock, simmer uncovered for 15 to 20 minutes, stirring occasionally. When vegetables are well cooked, turn off heat and leave to cool slightly. Add curry powder and evaporated milk and use a hand-held blender to purée, ensuring smooth consistency. Return to heat, stir constantly until soup heated to just before boiling point. Serve garnished with parsley.

Serves 4   * See recipe hints p.132

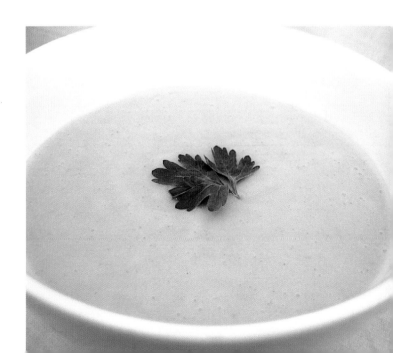

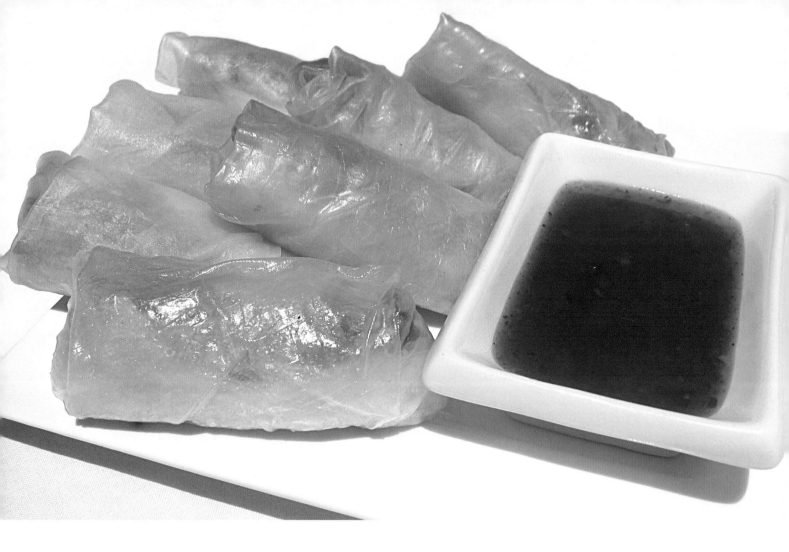

RICEPAPER ROLLS WITH DIPPING SAUCE

100g fine dried rice vermicelli noodles
200g chicken thigh fillet, cut into very fine strips
1/4 cup (65ml) prepared gluten free sweet chilli sauce
1 packet round ricepaper sheets (22cm diam.)
1 cup (35g) lettuce, finely shredded
1 small (120g) carrot, cut into fine julienne strips, 3 cm long
1/2 cup fresh coriander, finely chopped
1/2 cup (125ml) prepared gluten free sweet chilli sauce, extra

Fill a large bowl with hot water. Break the rice noodles up into 10cm pieces. Soak for 4 to 5 minutes or until tender, then rinse under cold water and drain well. Toss chicken strips in prepared chilli sauce in frying pan over medium heat for 1 to 2 minutes. Set aside.

Fill a large round flat dish (e.g. flan dish) with hot water. Place a ricepaper sheet in water and soak for approximately 1 minute, or until softened. Blot dry on paper towel or a clean tea towel. Place a small spoonful of pre-soaked noodles, 1 tablespoon of shredded lettuce, 2 or 3 pieces of carrot and some chicken strips in a line approximately 4 to 5cm long, on the bottom third of the ricepaper sheet. Top with a sprinkle of chopped coriander. Roll over once and fold in edges. Continue to roll up tightly. Arrange on a platter covered with moist cloth until all rolls prepared. Serve with extra sweet chilli sauce for dipping. Cover with plastic wrap and refrigerate if not serving immediately.

Makes 25

SAVOURY PIKELET STARTERS

1/3 cup (55g) rice flour
1/4 cup (60g) potato flour •
1/4 cup (50g) corn flour
1/4 tsp bicarb soda
1 egg, beaten
2/3 cup (165ml) reduced fat milk •
1 Tbsp butter, melted
salt, freshly ground black pepper to taste
cooking spray

4 Tbsp prepared gluten free olive tapenade (see p. 22)
4 Tbsp prepared gluten free sun-dried tomato spread (see p. 22)
4 Tbsp prepared gluten free pesto (see p. 22)

Sift flours and bicarb soda into a large bowl. Make a well in the centre, add beaten egg and milk. Blend well to make a smooth batter. Stir in melted butter and season with salt and pepper. Set aside for 10 minutes.

Heat a large frying pan over medium heat and spray with cooking spray. Spoon 1 to 2 tablespoons of batter into the frying pan, forming small pikelets. Cook for 1 minute each side or until light golden brown and just cooked through. Transfer to plate and cover to keep warm. Continue until all the batter is used. Top each pikelet with a small spoonful of prepared toppings. Serve warm.

Makes 30   • • See recipe hints p.132

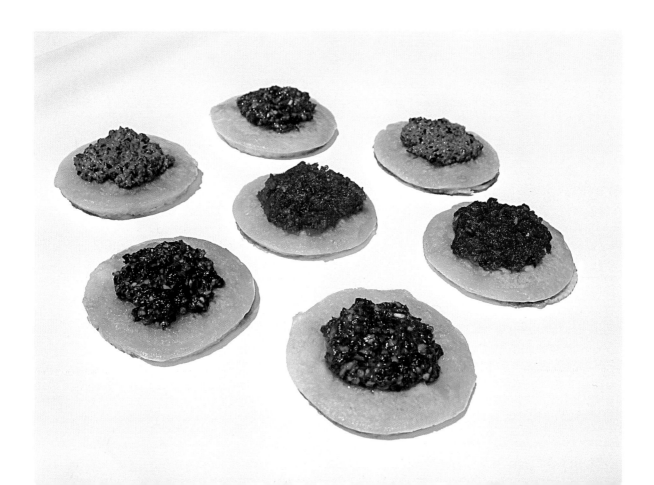

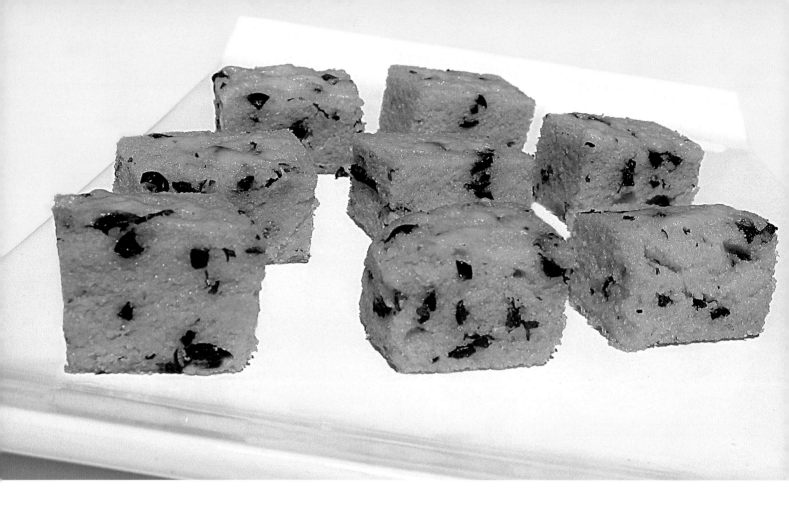

CHEESE & OLIVE POLENTA FINGERS

3 cups (750ml) gluten free chicken stock
1 cup (200g) instant polenta
1/3 cup (35g) pitted black olives, finely chopped
1/4 cup (30g) parmesan cheese, grated
1 1/2 Tbsp (30g) butter
1/4 cup fresh parsley, chopped
1/4 cup (30g) parmesan cheese, grated, extra

Bring chicken stock to the boil in a medium-sized saucepan. Pour in instant polenta, and cook over medium heat for 3 to 5 minutes, stirring constantly. Mixture should become very thick. Add olives, cheese, butter and parsley. Mix through until well combined. Pour into a greaseproof paper-lined 15cm x 15cm baking dish. Smooth the surface, cool slightly and then refrigerate for 1 hour.

Pre-heat oven to 180°C. Turn polenta out onto a chopping board, and cut into 3cm x 2cm fingers. Place on greased baking tray. Sprinkle each finger with extra grated parmesan cheese and bake in pre-heated oven for 10 to 15 minutes or cheese melted and fingers begin to turn golden brown. Serve warm.

Makes 30

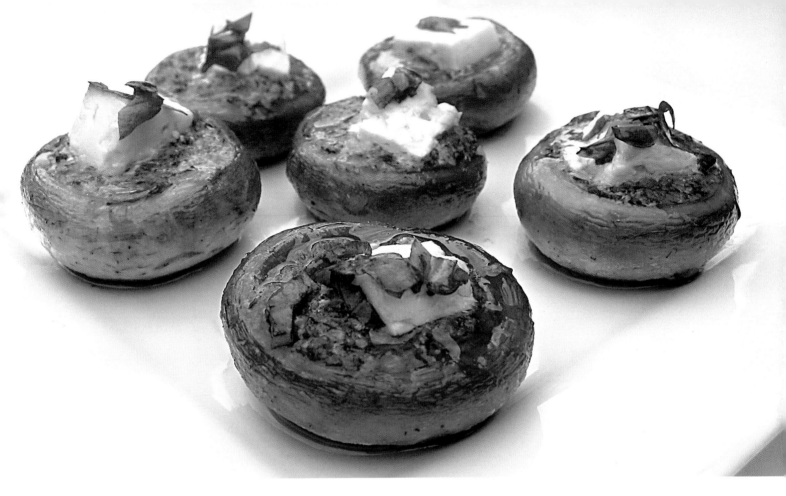

PESTO AND FETTA MUSHROOMS

15 medium (300g) button mushrooms
1/3 cup gluten free prepared pesto (see p. 22)
150g fetta cheese, cut into 1cm cubes
4 leaves fresh basil, chopped

Pre-heat oven to 180°C. Use a damp cloth to wipe clean the outer skin of each mushroom.
Remove stem and place on greased baking tray. Fill each mushroom with 1/2-1 teaspoon of
prepared pesto, and top with cube of fetta cheese. Bake in pre-heated oven for 5 to 10 minutes,
or until fetta begins to turn golden brown. Remove from oven, cover with aluminium foil for
2 minutes. Mushrooms will sweat and become soft. Remove foil. Sprinkle chopped basil to
garnish. Serve warm.

Makes 15

DIM SIMS

500g pork mince
150g prawn meat, finely chopped
2/3 cup (90g) bamboo shoots, finely chopped
1 cup (90g) savoy or Chinese cabbage, finely chopped
1 egg, lightly beaten
2 Tbsp gluten free soy sauce
2 tsp sesame oil
1 large clove garlic, crushed
11/2 tsp fresh ginger, finely grated
1 Tbsp gluten free cornflour
16cm diameter round ricepaper sheets
cooking string
polyunsaturated vegetable oil

Pre-heat oven to 150°C. Combine pork mince, prawn meat, bamboo shoots and cabbage in a bowl. In a small bowl, combine egg, soy sauce, oil, garlic, ginger and cornflour and mix well. Pour sauce over meat mixture and mix until well combined. Fill a large round flat dish (e.g. flan dish) with hot water. Place a ricepaper sheet in water and soak for approximately 1 minute, or until softened. Blot dry on paper towel or clean tea towel. Place 11/2 tablespoons of meat mixture in the centre of each soaked ricepaper sheet. Gather ricepaper sheet up in the middle, and tie in a bow tie with cooking string. Repeat this process until all filling used.

Heat oil in deep fryer to 180°C (or heat a large saucepan of oil over medium-low heat. Use a thermometer if you have one). Deep fry 4 to 5 dim sims at a time for 5 minutes. You may wish to commence frying whilst still making the remainder of the dim sims. When cooked, remove dim sims from oil with slotted spoon and drain on paper towel. Untie bow and remove string. Keep warm in oven until all cooked.

Hint: Although these are a little fiddly, they are worth the effort.

Makes 24

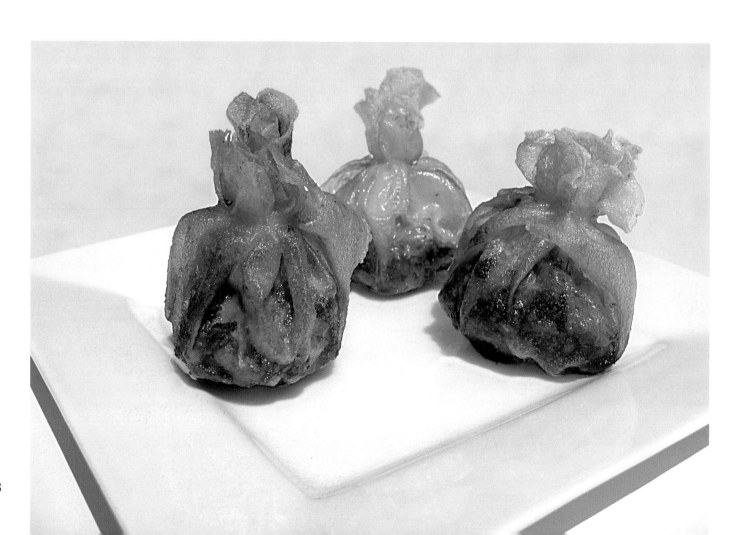

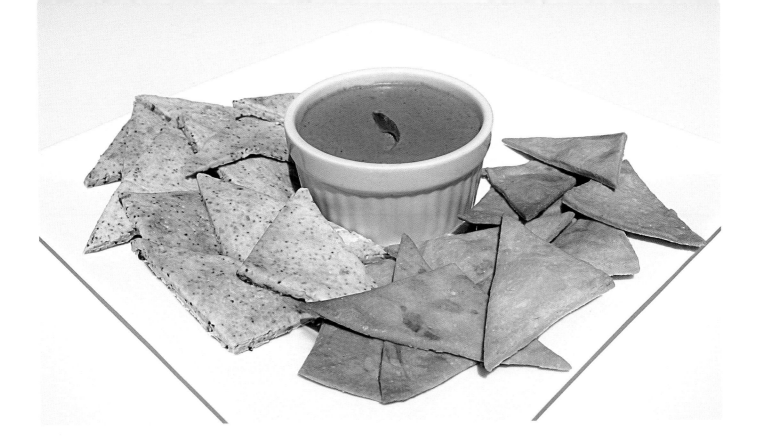

CRACKED PEPPER PATÉ

2 cloves garlic, crushed
1 large onion, cut into 1cm-thick strips
1 tsp fresh sage, chopped
125g butter
500g chicken livers
1 Tbsp ground black pepper
1/2 cup (125ml) cream
50g butter, melted, extra
sage leaves, extra for decoration

In a medium saucepan over medium heat, cook garlic, onions and sage in butter for 7 to 8 minutes, stirring regularly. Add livers, cook until browned, then remove from heat. Using a fork, remove all onion strips from pan and discard. Stir through ground pepper and cream. Purée with hand-held blender or in food processor until smooth. Finally, add additional melted butter and blend until well combined. Pour into 1/2 cup serving pots, and top with sage leaf. Cover, then refrigerate for 3 hours or until set.

SAVOURY WAFERS

1 cup (130g) fine rice flour •
40g butter (for a flakier wafer, increase butter to 50g)
1/4 tsp salt
1 egg, lightly beaten
1 Tbsp water
2 Tbsp milk

Pre-heat oven to 180°C. Grease two baking trays.
Rub butter into flour until mixture resembles fine breadcrumbs. Add flavourings of choice, mix well. Finally add egg and water. Combine to form a dough, and knead lightly. Roll to 2mm thickness between two sheets of baking paper.
Cut into triangles and place on baking trays. Brush with milk, and bake in pre-heated oven for 15 minutes. Allow to cool for 2 minutes on baking tray before transferring to wire rack to cool completely.

Flavour variations:
Three seed: Add 2 Tbsp sesame seeds, 1 Tbsp sunflower seeds, 2 tsp poppy seeds
Parmesan and thyme: Add 2 Tbsp parmesan cheese and 1 tsp chopped fresh thyme

• See recipe hints p.132

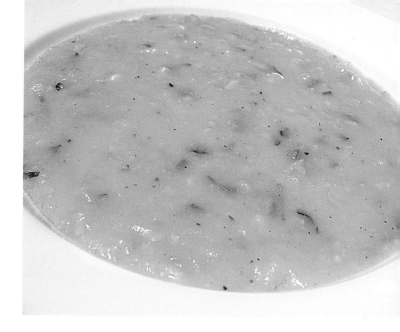

RED LENTIL AND SWEET POTATO SOUP

2 large (1200g) sweet potatoes (kumara), peeled
8 cups (2L) gluten free vegetable stock
1 cup (200g) dried split red lentils
4 Tbsp fresh coriander, chopped (more to taste)
2 Tbsp fresh basil, chopped
salt, freshly ground black pepper to taste

Cut sweet potatoes into 2cm pieces. In a large saucepan, bring vegetable stock to the boil. Add sweet potato, red lentils and chopped coriander. Turn down heat to low, and cook, covered, for 40 minutes, stirring occasionally. Remove from heat, and use hand blender to purée until smooth in consistency. Stir through chopped basil and additional coriander if desired. Add salt and pepper to taste.

Hint: This soup thickens on standing. You may thin it down by adding milk or water as desired.

Serves 4

POTATO AND SWEETCORN SOUP

400g lean rindless bacon, diced
3 medium (540g) potatoes, peeled, diced
2 small onions, whole, peeled
3 Tbsp butter
4 Tbsp gluten free cornflour
8 cups (2L) strong gluten free chicken stock
2 x 440g can gluten free creamed corn
1/2 tsp mustard powder
1/2 tsp fresh thyme, chopped
1 Tbsp fresh parsley, chopped
salt, freshly ground black pepper to taste

In a large heavy-based saucepan over medium heat, sauté diced bacon, potatoes and whole onions in butter. Stir regularly until bacon is browned. Mix cornflour with a little chicken stock to form a paste. Add remaining chicken stock slowly to cornflour paste, mixing well to ensure smooth in consistency. Pour over bacon and potato. Cook uncovered over medium heat for 15 minutes, stirring occasionally. Remove from heat, and remove whole onions, discard. Purée with hand-held blender until even in consistency, then stir through creamed corn, mustard, thyme and parsley. Taste, season with salt and pepper.

Serves 4

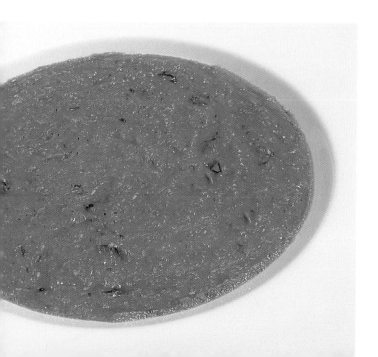

CALIFORNIA ROLLS

2 1/2 cups (550g) short grain (Koshikari) rice
4 cups (1000ml) water
1/3 cup (85ml) sushi vinegar
1 Tbsp caster sugar
1/2 tsp salt
6 sheets nori (seaweed paper)
gluten free wasabi paste for serving

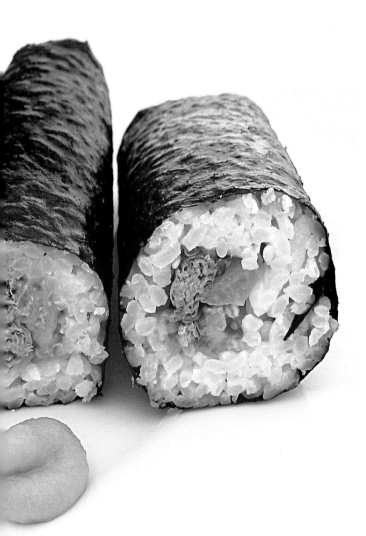

Place rice and water in large saucepan. Cook, covered, over medium-low heat for 8 minutes. Remove from heat, keep lid on saucepan, and allow to stand for 10 minutes. Combine vinegar, sugar and salt in small bowl. Stir until sugar dissolved. Transfer rice into a large mixing bowl; add vinegar mix, stirring gently through to make rice grains slightly sticky but still separated. Keep warm, cover with damp tea towel. Do not refrigerate.

Place single sheet of nori on top of a sheet of greaseproof paper, on a flat surface (or use sushi mats if you have them). Spread 1 cup of cooked rice, 3mm thick, over closest 2/3 of nori sheet. Place strips of chosen filling on prepared rice bed, in a line 11/2 cm from front edge of nori. Begin to roll sushi, commencing with rice-prepared end. Pick up greaseproof paper, together with prepared nori and begin to turn into itself. Keep tight by rolling firmly against the greaseproof paper. After completing 3/4 of a turn, pack extra rice along edge of filling, so that when full turn is completed, the filling will be centred in the rice. Continue the turn until all of the nori is rolled. Do not include greaseproof paper/mat in the full turn, separate it from the nori. Repeat for remaining sheets. Refrigerate for 1 hour, and then slice each roll in half with serrated knife. Serve with wasabi paste.

Filling suggestions

Tuna: 210g can tuna mixed with 2 Tbsp gluten free mayonnaise, shredded lettuce
Spinach and avocado: 3 cups wilted baby spinach leaves, 1 avocado (240g) sliced, egg omelette strips, gluten free mayonnaise
Prawn and avocado: 12 medium (350g) cooked peeled prawns, 1 avocado, toasted sesame seeds
Vegetarian: avocado strips, fried bean curd, julienne sliced carrot sticks, shredded lettuce, cucumber strips, gluten free mayonnaise, sesame seeds
Smoked salmon: 200g smoked salmon, 1 avocado sliced, cucumber strips, gluten free mayonnaise

Makes 12

OLIVE TAPENADE

1 cup (140g) pitted black olives
40g anchovy fillets, drained
2 Tbsp gluten free whole egg mayonnaise
1 clove garlic, crushed
2 tsp lemon juice
1 Tbsp olive oil

Place olives, anchovies, mayonnaise, garlic, lemon juice and olive oil into the bowl of a food processor. Process until just blended.

SALSA VERDE

1 bunch parsley, washed, dried
3 anchovy fillets, drained
2 tsp capers, drained
2 cloves garlic, crushed
1/2 cup (125ml) olive oil
2 Tbsp lemon juice (approx.)
salt, freshly ground black pepper

Place washed parsley, anchovies, capers and garlic into the bowl of a food processor. Process until well combined. Gradually add the olive oil to the processor until well blended. Add lemon juice, salt and pepper according to personal flavour preference.

BASIL PESTO

3 cups (100g) firmly packed fresh basil leaves
1 large clove garlic, crushed
1/3 cup (65ml) olive oil
1/3 cup (55g) pine nuts (or cashew nuts)
1/3 cup (40g) parmesan cheese, grated
salt, freshly ground black pepper

Place washed basil, garlic, oil, nuts and cheese into the bowl of a food processor. Process until well combined. Season with salt and pepper. Add more oil for a more liquid pesto if desired.

SUN-DRIED TOMATO SPREAD

1 cup (210g) sun-dried tomatoes, roughly chopped, retain o
1/4 cup fresh parsley leaves, roughly chopped
2 Tbsp cream cheese
2 cloves garlic, crushed
1/4 cup (65ml) olive oil
salt, freshly ground black pepper

Place the sun-dried tomatoes, parsley, cream cheese, and garlic in the bowl of a food processor. Process until well combined. Gradually add the olive oil to the processor until the mixture is almost smooth. Season with salt and pepper.

Hint: Store all in an airtight container in the refrigerator until required

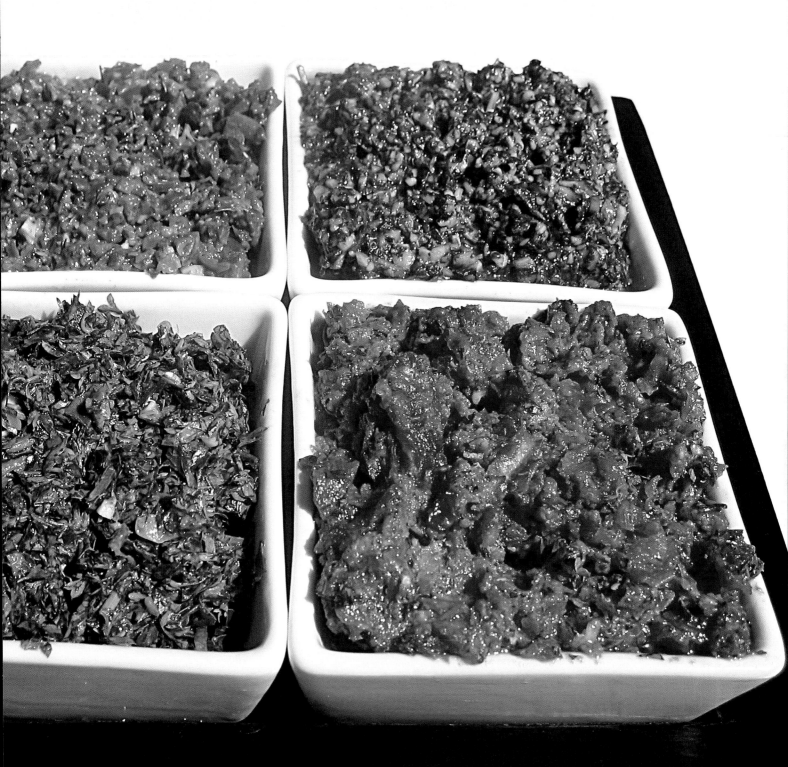

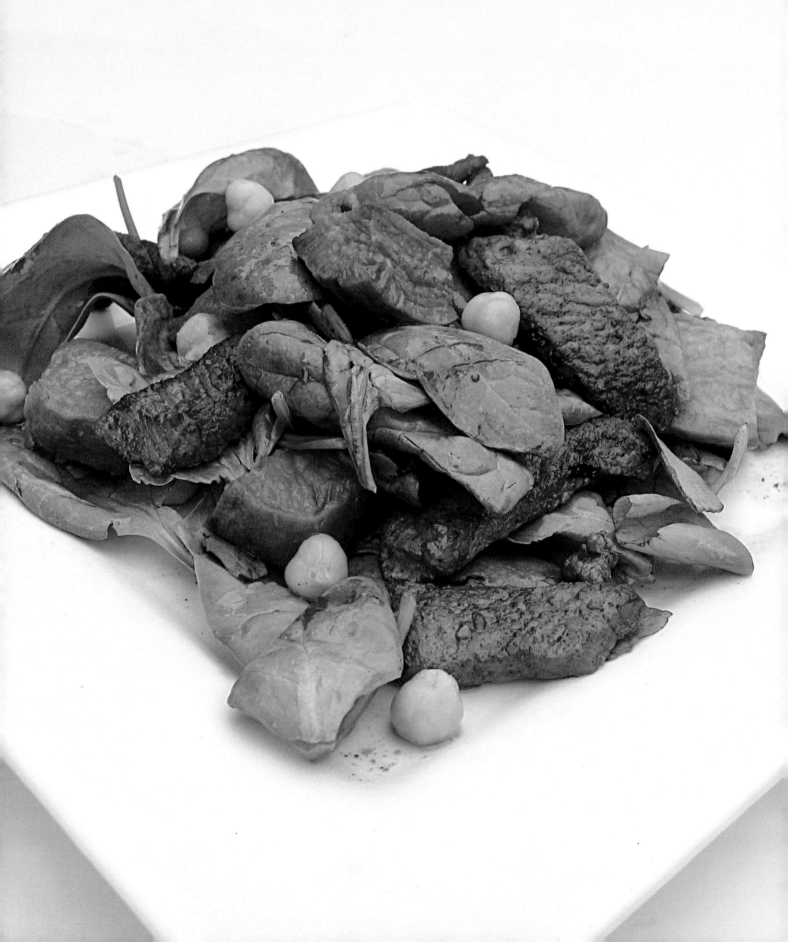

lights

BARBECUED SALT AND PEPPER CALAMARI

8 medium (1000g) calamari hoods (squid tubes)
3 Tbsp olive oil
2 cloves garlic, crushed
1/2 tsp salt
freshly ground black pepper

Fresh Garden Salad
4 1/2 cups (150g) lettuce leaves, roughly chopped
1/2 (200g) continental cucumber, diced
1 avocado (240g), sliced
2 sticks (180g) celery, thinly sliced
1/2 (150g) green capsicum, diced
1 cup (70g) snow pea sprouts

Dressing
1/4 cup (65ml) olive oil
3 Tbsp lemon juice
1/2 clove garlic, crushed
1/2 tsp brown sugar
salt

Rinse calamari hoods and then cut them into quarters. With a sharp knife, score calamari pieces in a 1cm criss-cross action, halfway through. This will ensure the calamari will curl when cooked. Do not cut all the way through. Combine olive oil, garlic, salt and pepper together in a large bowl. Toss calamari pieces in oil mix, cover, refrigerate for 3 to 4 hours.

Prepare salad: combine lettuce, cucumber, avocado, celery, capsicum and sprouts in a large salad bowl. Distribute over four serving dishes. Prepare dressing: combine olive oil, lemon juice, garlic, sugar and salt in a jar. Shake well to combine. Set aside.

Remove calamari from refrigerator and cook pieces over high heat on barbecue, chargrill or in frying pan for 3 to 4 minutes, or until chargrilled in appearance. Shake salad dressing and drizzle over prepared salad plates. Arrange cooked calamari on top. Serve while calamari warm.

Serves 4

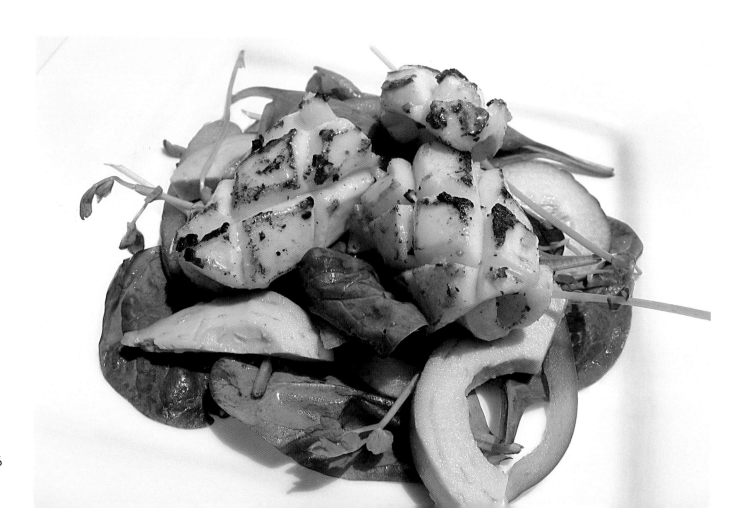

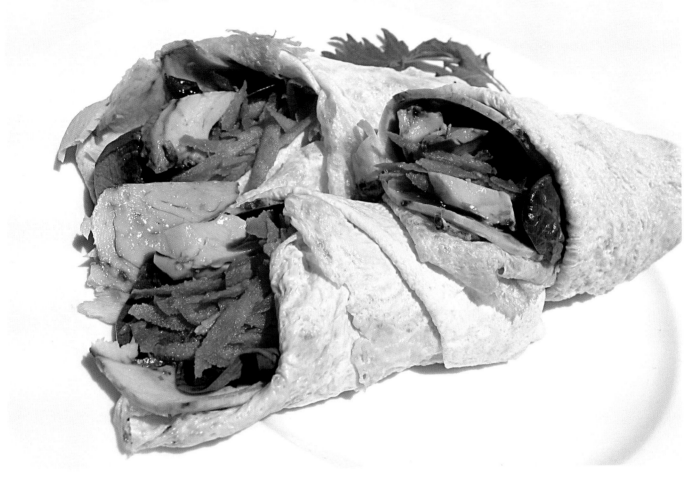

OMELETTE WRAPS

6 eggs
6 thin slices (100g) turkey breast
3 tsp cranberry sauce
1 medium (240g) avocado, sliced
2 cups (70g) baby spinach leaves, washed
1 medium (140g) tomato, sliced
1/2 cup (60g) carrot, grated

Heat small non-stick frying pan over medium heat and spray with cooking spray. Crack one egg into small bowl, whisk with fork. Pour egg into hot frying pan, rolling frying pan to ensure egg is spread thin and evenly over the pan, approximately 12cm in diameter. Cook for 30 seconds to 1 minute, then flip with egg lifter, being careful not to break omelette. (Alternatively if you have a flat sandwich press, cook omelette in this, it is quick and easy). Set aside on plate. Repeat until all six omelettes formed, set aside to cool.

Place egg omelette on flat surface. Lay one slice of turkey breast on top half of omelette, and top with 1/2 teaspoon of cranberry sauce and 1/6 avocado. Add baby spinach leaves, sliced tomato and sprinkle of grated carrot. Fold bottom third of omelette base up into centre of omelette. Roll from left to right, encasing all contents in the wrap. Serve immediately or cover and refrigerate.

Alternative filling suggestions:
• Smoked salmon, cream cheese, capers and cracked pepper.
• Chicken with curried gluten free mayonnaise.
• Shredded ham, sliced beetroot, tomato and avocado.

Makes 6

SMOKED CHICKEN SALAD WITH WALNUT DRESSING

1/2 cup gluten free whole egg mayonnaise
1/2 tsp gluten free soy sauce
2 Tbsp lemon juice
1/4 cup (35g) walnuts, finely chopped
4 cups (140g) baby cos lettuce leaves
1 x 410g can beetroot wedges, drained, dried on paper towel
1/2 cup alfalfa sprouts
4 hard boiled eggs, cut in quarters
1 medium (240g) avocado, sliced
500g smoked chicken, sliced

In a small bowl, combine mayonnaise, soy sauce, lemon juice and walnuts. Set aside.

Rinse lettuce leaves, drain, and transfer to a large salad bowl. Pour over prepared dressing, toss gently to coat. Distribute between four bowls. Arrange drained beetroot, sprouts, eggs and avocado neatly on lettuce bed. Finally top with sliced smoked chicken.

Serves 4

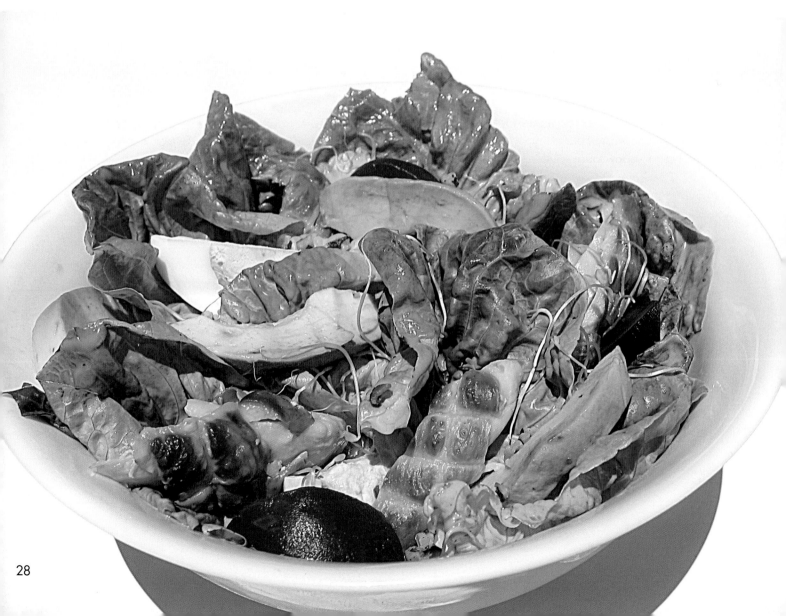

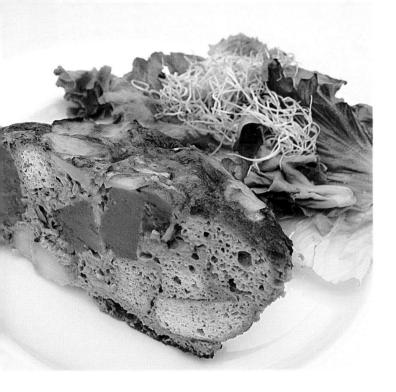

WASABI VEGETABLE FRITTATA

1 medium (180g) potato, cut into 1cm cubes
200g pumpkin, peeled, cut into 1cm cubes
2 Tbsp gluten free wasabi paste
2 Tbsp gluten free soy sauce
1/2 cup (125ml) milk •
6 eggs, lightly beaten
salt, freshly ground black pepper to taste
1 medium (150g) zucchini, grated
100g fried tofu squares, cut into 1cm cubes

Pre-heat oven to 170°C. Grease 16cm x 16cm baking dish. Add cubed potato and pumpkin to saucepan of boiling water. Cook over medium heat until just tender. In large mixing bowl, mix wasabi paste and soy sauce together. Slowly add milk, eggs, salt and pepper to taste, blend well. Stir in cooked potato and pumpkin, grated zucchini and tofu. Pour mixture into greased baking dish. Bake in pre-heated oven for 25 to 30 minutes or until golden brown. Let stand for 5 minutes before cutting into wedges. May be served warm or cool.

Serves 8   • See recipe hints p.132

ZUCCHINI SLICE

2 large (500g) zucchini, grated
10 rashers (200g) rindless bacon, diced
11/2 cups (150g) tasty cheese, grated
1/2 cup (85g) rice flour
1/4 cup (35g) gluten free cornflour
2 Tbsp canola oil
6 eggs, lightly beaten
salt, freshly ground black pepper to taste

Pre-heat oven to 170°C. Combine zucchini, bacon, cheese, flours, oil, eggs and seasonings in a large bowl. Pour into a greased shallow baking tray (16 x 26cm) and bake in pre-heated oven for 20 to 25 minutes, or until firm and golden brown. Let stand for 5 minutes before slicing.

Serves 6

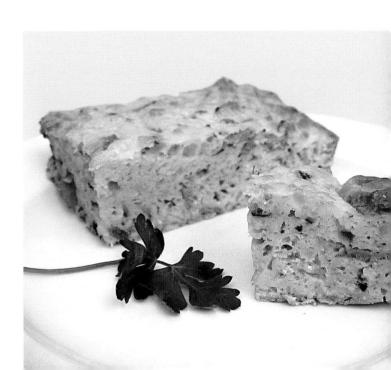

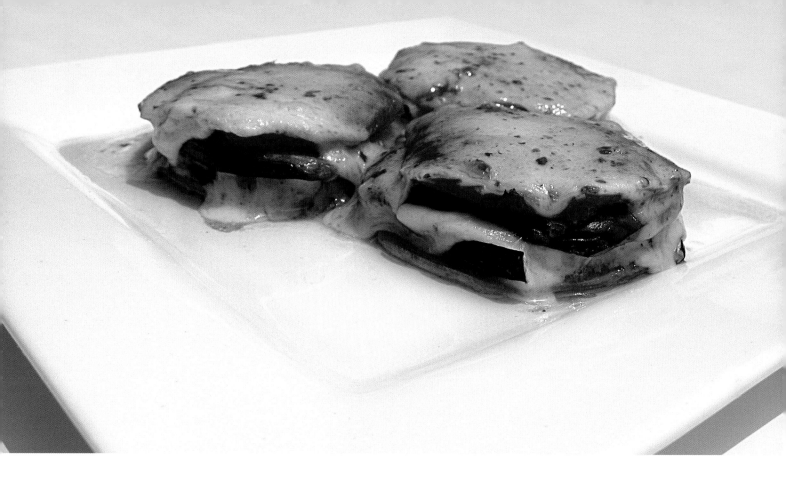

ROASTED VEGETABLE STACK

1 large (500g) eggplant, sliced into 5mm-thick pieces
2 large zucchinis (500g), sliced lengthways into
   5mm-thick pieces
1 small wide (250g) orange sweet potato, peeled,
   sliced into 5mm-thick pieces
1 medium (300g) red capsicum, cut into 5cm-wide strips
1 Tbsp olive oil
3/4 cup (90g) parmesan cheese, grated
320g mozzarella cheese, thinly sliced
1/2 cup prepared gluten free basil pesto (see p. 22)
salt, freshly ground black pepper to taste

Pre-heat oven to 170°C. Place layers of eggplant,
zucchini, sweet potato and capsicum on baking trays.
Brush with a little olive oil, and bake in pre-heated oven
for 15 to 20 minutes or until vegetables tender.

On a large baking tray lined with baking paper, place
slices of roasted sweet potato. Sprinkle each slice with 1 to 2
tablespoons parmesan cheese. Top with zucchini slice and
1/2 of the mozzarella. Spread with 1/3 of the pesto. Then top
with layer of eggplant, and sprinkle with 1 to 2 tablespoons
of parmesan cheese. Top with a layer of capsicum and
sliced mozzarella cheese. Spread remaining pesto on top.
Bake in pre-heated oven for 10 to 15 minutes until the stack
is heated through.

Hint: For round vegetable stacks, use a scone or pastry cutter
to cut vegetables to shape prior to forming stacks.

Serves 4

AUSSIE MEAT PIE

Pastry
1 cup (130g) fine rice flour •
1/2 cup (75g) gluten free cornflour
1/2 cup (45g) soy flour •
1 tsp xanthan gum (optional) •
160g butter
6 Tbsp (120ml) iced water

Filling
500g lean beef mince
1/2 smalll (60g) carrot, peeled, finely grated
1/2 cup (70g) gluten free gravy powder
1 cup (250ml) water
1/4 tsp gluten free "Vegemite ™" (optional)
1 egg, lightly beaten

Pastry: Pre-heat oven to 170°C. Grease four 12cm diameter individual pie dishes. Sift flours and xanthan gum three times into a bowl. Combine sifted flours and butter in food processor. Process until it resembles fine breadcrumbs. While the motor is running, add iced water (tablespoon at a time) to allow mixture to form soft dough. Knead on gluten-free corn-floured bench. Wrap in plastic wrap and refrigerate for 30 minutes before rolling to use. Roll pastry 1 to 2mm thick between two sheets of non-stick baking paper. Place pie dish upside down onto pastry, and use a knife to cut around edge. Cut four circles. Also cut four larger circles using a 14cm saucer plate. Place the larger pastry circles into greased pie dishes, trim edges to neaten. Bake in pre-heated oven for 7 to 8 minutes or until lightly browned. Reserve small pastry circles for tops.

Filling: In a medium saucepan, combine mince, carrot, gravy powder, water and "vegemite". Cook over medium heat until mince is browned and in a thick gravy. Place 1/4 of meat mixture into cooked pie base. Place reserved pastry circle on top, seal edges. Brush pie top with egg, bake in pre-heated oven for 10 to 15 minutes or until golden brown. Allow to cool in tins for 5 minutes then transfer to wire rack to cool completely.

Makes 4   • See recipe hints p.132

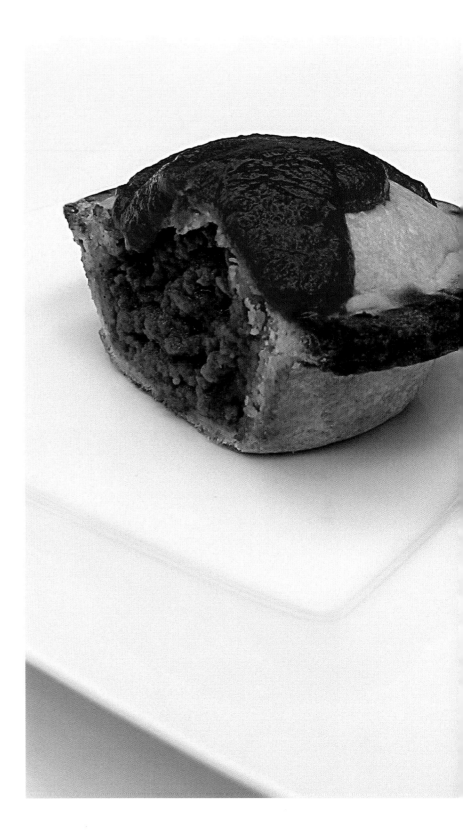

LIGHT AND FRESH OMELETTE

1 Tbsp canola oil
4 eggs
1 Tbsp fresh basil, chopped
1 Tbsp fresh parsley, chopped
salt, freshly ground black pepper to taste
1/2 cup (70g) lean chicken, cooked, diced
1/2 cup baby spinach leaves
1/2 medium (150g) red capsicum, diced
1/4 cup (40g) button mushrooms, sliced
3 Tbsp tasty cheese, grated

Heat oil in a small frying pan over medium heat. Whisk 2 eggs, basil, parsley, salt and pepper in medium mixing bowl. Add to pan and cook until almost set on top. Use egg lifter carefully at edges, and shake omelette loose on the pan. Top with half of all toppings evenly over one half of omelette. Fold omelette in half to encase toppings. Continue to heat until cooked through.

Repeat for second omelette, or alternatively, cook all eggs together in larger frying pan and cut large omelette in half prior to serving.

Serves 2

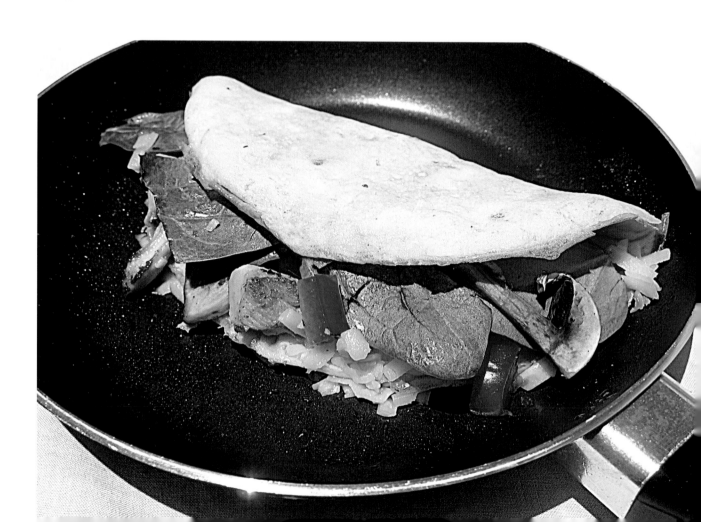

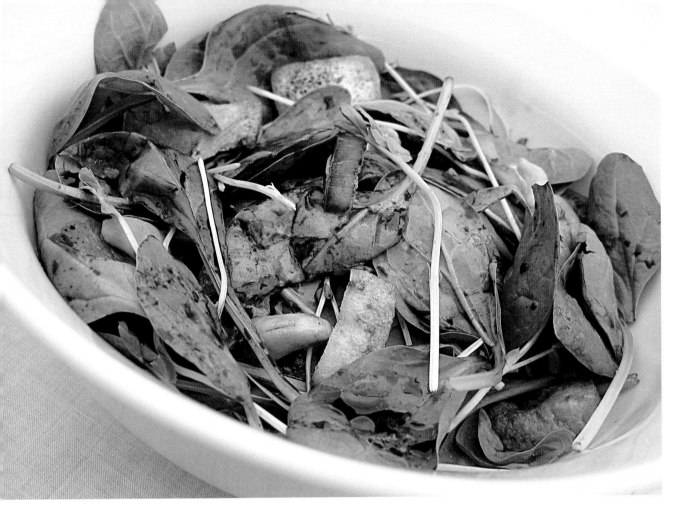

SPINACH TOFU SALAD

3 Tbsp (60ml) gluten free soy sauce
3 Tbsp (60ml) lemon juice
1 Tbsp sushi vinegar
3 Tbsp brown sugar
3 Tbsp sesame oil
9 cups (300g) baby spinach leaves
1 1/2 cups (105g) snow pea sprouts
1 medium (300g) green capsicum, sliced into 2cm lengths
400g fried tofu puffs (bean curd), cubed
1 cup (170g) cashews

In a small mixing bowl, combine soy sauce, lemon juice, sushi vinegar, sugar and sesame oil. Set aside.

In a large mixing bowl, toss spinach, snow pea sprouts, capsicum, tofu and cashews until well combined. Distribute over four serving bowls. Drizzle prepared dressing over salads.

Serves 4

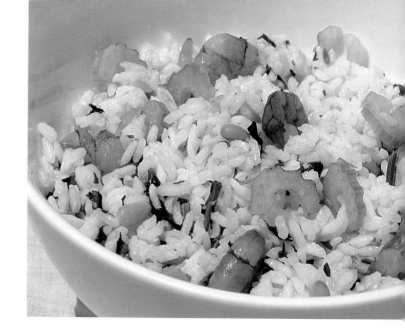

SCRAMBLED EGGS

10 eggs
3/4 cup (190ml) reduced fat cream
salt, freshly ground black pepper, to taste
2 Tbsp butter

Whisk eggs and cream together well in a large bowl. Season with salt and pepper. Melt butter in a medium sized frying pan over low heat. Add the egg mixture to the frying pan. Use a wooden spoon to push the egg mixture around edges and into the middle of the pan, every ten seconds to prevent sticking. Cook for approximately 5 minutes or until almost all the egg mixture is cooked. Ensure the mixture is still creamy and slightly runny.

Flavour variation: Stir in 100g thinly sliced smoked salmon, just before serving.

Serves 4

PRAWN RICE SALAD

1 cup (220g) long grain rice
6 cups (1 1/2L) gluten free vegetable stock
2 tsp sesame oil
2 sticks (180g) celery
2/3 cup (110g) pine nuts
500g cooked, peeled prawns
1/2 cup fresh parsley, chopped
4 Tbsp sesame oil, extra
1 1/2 Tbsp lemon rind, finely grated
1/4 cup (65ml) lemon juice

Cook rice in vegetable stock until tender. Rinse well, drain and set aside. In a large frying pan, heat sesame oil and sauté celery and pine nuts over medium heat until celery is tender and pine nuts are golden brown. Add cooked prawns and rice, parsley, sesame oil, lemon rind and juice. Stir until well combined, heating through. May be served warm or at room temperature.

Serves 4

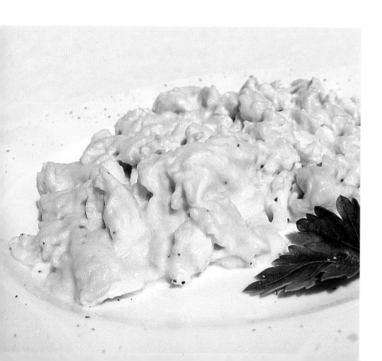

CHICKPEA AND ROASTED SWEET POTATO SALAD

2 medium (800g) sweet potatoes, peeled, cut into 2cm cubes
olive oil
400g lean lamb steaks, cut into strips
2 Tbsp gluten free Middle Eastern spices
6 cups (200g) baby spinach leaves
1 x 425g can chickpeas, drained
2 tsp gluten free Middle Eastern spices, extra

Pre-heat oven to 180°C. Place sweet potato cubes in a baking dish and brush with olive oil. Roast in oven for 30 minutes or until cooked and golden brown. Allow to cool. Heat a little olive oil and spices in a frying pan over medium-low heat for 1 minute to develop flavour. Add lamb strips, stir through spices to coat well. Cook until just browned and then remove from heat. In a large bowl, combine baby spinach leaves, sweet potato and chickpeas. Distribute over four serving plates. Top with cooked lamb and pan juices. Sprinkle salad with additional spices and drizzle with olive oil to taste.

Serves 4

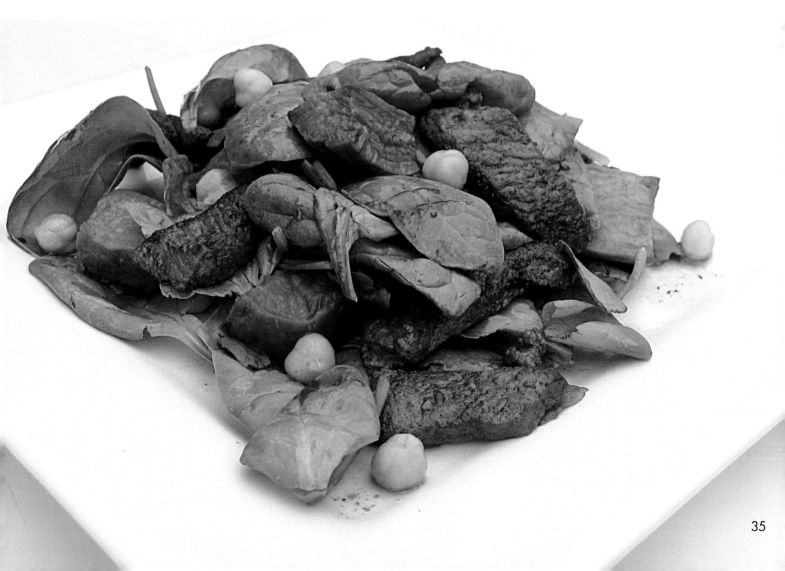

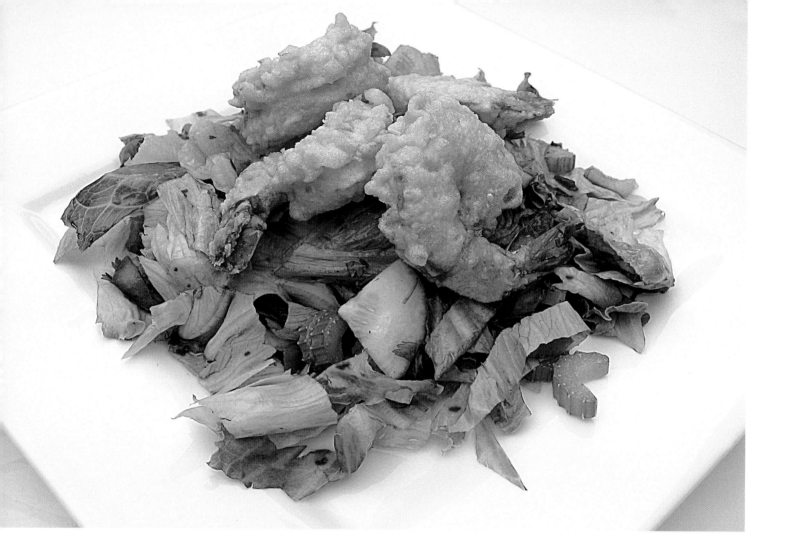

SESAME PRAWNS WITH CORIANDER SALAD

1 egg
1 cup (145g) gluten free cornflour
2/3 cup (125ml) water
3 Tbsp sesame seeds, toasted
sunflower oil for deep frying
16 (220g) green prawns, shelled, tails intact
1/4 cup (35g) gluten free cornflour, extra

In a medium mixing bowl, combine egg, cornflour, water and sesame seeds. Mix until well combined and smooth in consistency. Refrigerate for 30 minutes.

Heat oil in a deep fryer to 180°C, or in large saucepan over medium-low heat (use a thermometer if you have one). Toss prawns in extra cornflour, then into batter mix, and then immediately into heated oil. Cook for 3 to 4 minutes or until batter crispy.

Coriander Salad
5 cups (150g) lettuce leaves, roughly chopped
1/2 (200g) continental cucumber, diced
2 sticks (160g) celery, thinly sliced
1/2 (150g) green capsicum, diced
1/2 cup fresh coriander, chopped
1 Tbsp fresh mint leaves, finely chopped
2 Tbsp lemon juice
1 Tbsp sushi vinegar
2 tsp sugar
1/2 small chilli, deseeded, finely chopped (optional)

Combine lettuce, cucumber, celery, capsicum and coriander in a large salad bowl. In a small bowl, combine mint, lemon juice, vinegar, sugar and chilli paste. Pour over salad just before serving. Top with fried sesame prawns.

Serves 4

MEDITERRANEAN SLICE

6 medium (120g) button mushrooms, sliced
1 medium (150g) zucchini, halved and sliced
2 tomatoes (280g), chopped
2 tsp olive oil
1 Tbsp balsamic vinegar
1 tsp dried Italian mixed herbs
1 cup (100g) tasty cheese, grated
1/2 cup (60g) parmesan cheese, grated
1/2 cup (85g) rice flour
1/4 cup (35g) gluten free cornflour
2 Tbsp olive oil, extra
6 eggs, lightly beaten
salt, freshly ground black pepper to taste
1 tsp dried Italian mixed herbs, extra

Pre-heat oven to 170°C. In a non-stick frying pan, sauté mushrooms, zucchini and tomatoes in olive oil, balsamic vinegar and mixed herbs. Cook until soft, remove from heat. Combine cooked vegetables, cheeses, flours, extra oil, eggs, salt and pepper in a large bowl. Pour into a greased shallow baking tray (16cm x 26cm). Sprinkle additional Italian mixed herbs evenly over top of mixture. Bake in pre-heated oven for 20 to 25 minutes, or until firm and golden brown. Allow to stand for 5 minutes before cutting into slices.

Serves 6

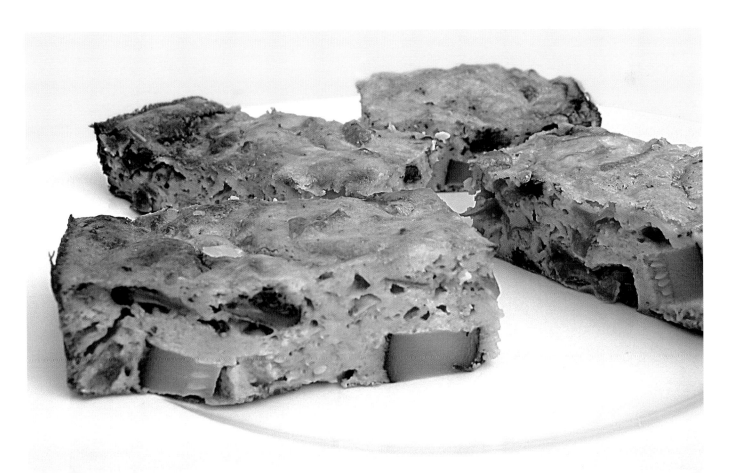

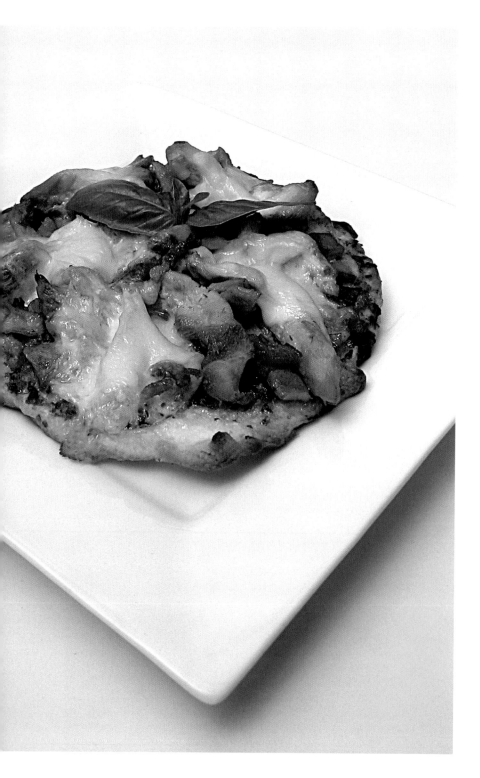

CHICKEN, BACON AND PESTO MINI PIZZAS

2 cups prepared gluten free bread mix
2 tsp olive oil
500g chicken breast fillets, thinly sliced
15 rashers (300g) lean bacon, sliced
2 cloves garlic, crushed
6 tsp prepared gluten free basil pesto
  (see p. 22)
6 large (250g) bocconcini cheese balls, sliced

Pre-heat oven to 120°C. Line two baking trays with greasproof paper. Make gluten free bread mix according to packet directions. Spoon 1/3 cup of bread mix onto greaseproof paper. Using the back of a metal spoon, spread the mix out to form a circle, 15cm diameter, approximately 3 to 5mm thick. Dip the spoon in water to assist in spreading if required. Repeat until six bases formed. Bake in pre-heated oven for 15 minutes, or until lightly browned. Remove from oven, turn temperature up to 180°C.

In a frying pan over medium heat, sauté chicken and bacon in oil until crispy. Remove from heat. Spread 1 teaspoon of pesto over base of pizza. Top with cooked bacon and chicken pieces, then with sliced bocconcici cheese. Bake in oven (on wire rack of oven to prevent base from becoming soggy) for 15 minutes or until cheese melted.

Serves 6

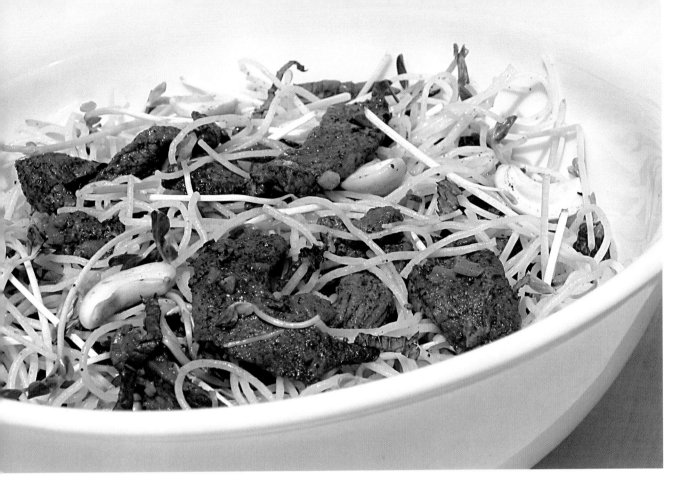

VIETNAMESE RICE NOODLE SALAD WITH MINT

400g beef rump steak, thinly sliced
3 cloves garlic, crushed
3 tsp Chinese five spice
3 Tbsp fish sauce
3 Tbsp sushi vinegar
2 tsp fresh ginger, grated
3 tsp brown sugar
250g dried rice vermicelli noodles
hot water
2 Tbsp sesame oil
1 cup (70g) snow pea sprouts
1/4 cup fresh mint, chopped
1/4 cup (40g) cashews

Cut rump steak into thin strips. In a medium bowl, mix garlic, Chinese five spice, fish sauce, vinegar, ginger and sugar. Add sliced steak, mix through until meat well coated in the marinade. Refrigerate for 3 hours.

Place rice noodles in heat-proof bowl, cover with boiling water. Let soak for 5 minutes, or until tender. Rinse under cold water, drain well.

Heat sesame oil in frying pan over medium heat. Add marinated steak and excess marinade, heat until just cooked through. Do not overcook to ensure meat remains tender. In a large bowl, combine noodles, snow pea sprouts, mint, cashews, cooked beef strips and meat juices. Distribute evenly over four bowls.

Serves 4

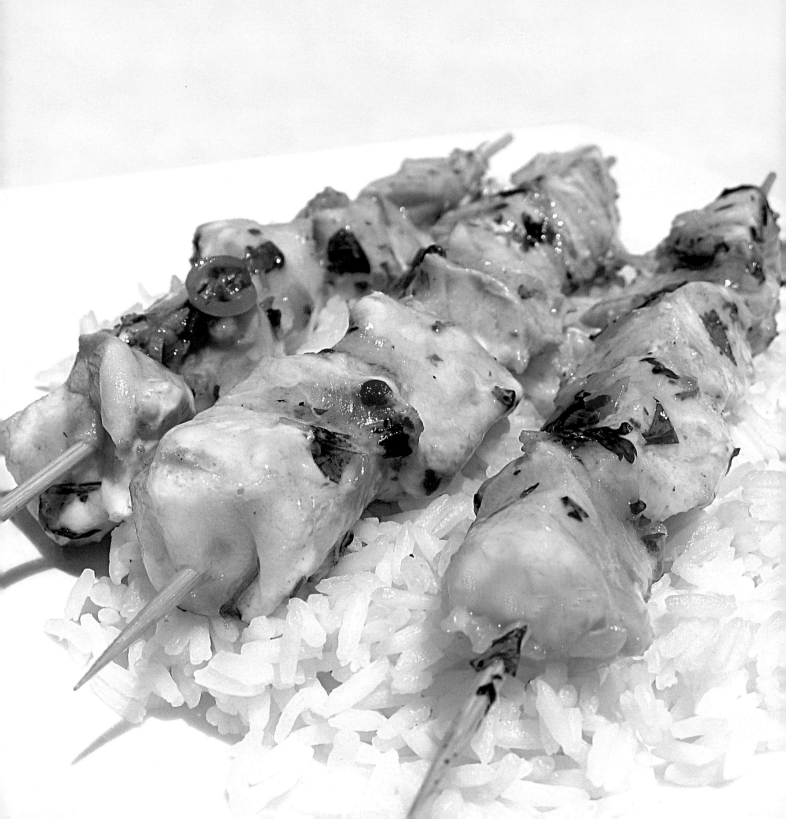

mains

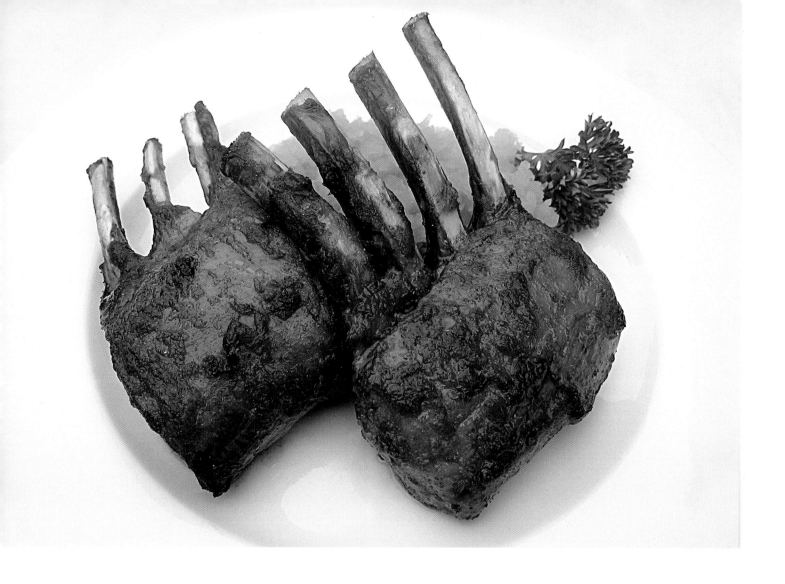

ROAST LAMB RACKS ON MASHED BUTTERED SWEDE

2 racks of 8 lamb cutlets (1kg), trimmed of fat
1¹/2 Tbsp (30g) butter, at room temperature
1 tsp ground cumin
salt, freshly ground black pepper to taste
2 large (650g) swede
1 Tbsp butter, extra
salt and pepper, extra

Pre-heat oven to 180°C. Combine butter, cumin, salt and pepper in a small bowl, rub over lamb cutlets. Place in baking dish and cook for 30 minutes or to liking. Remove from heat, cut each rack in half. Serve on bed of mashed buttered swede.

Mashed buttered swede: Peel swede and cut into 5cm chunks. Cook in boiling water until tender. Drain, then mash with butter and salt and pepper to taste.

Serves 4

CHICKEN WITH GOLDEN SAGE SAUCE

1 clove garlic, crushed
1 Tbsp olive oil
1 Tbsp lemon juice
salt, freshly ground pepper to taste
4 x 150g chicken breast fillets
80g butter
2 cloves garlic, crushed, extra
1/4 cup (25g) fresh parmesan cheese, grated
20 fresh sage leaves

Combine garlic, olive oil, lemon juice, salt and pepper in a small bowl. Add chicken breasts, toss until well coated. Refrigerate for 3 to 4 hours or overnight.

In a large frying pan over medium-low heat, pan-fry chicken fillets in 1 tablespoon of melted butter for 3 to 5 minutes each side, or until just cooked and golden brown. Melt remaining butter in a small frying pan and sauté extra garlic until golden brown. Add cheese and sage leaves, cook for 1 minute, or until sage leaves softened. Pour over chicken.

Serves 4

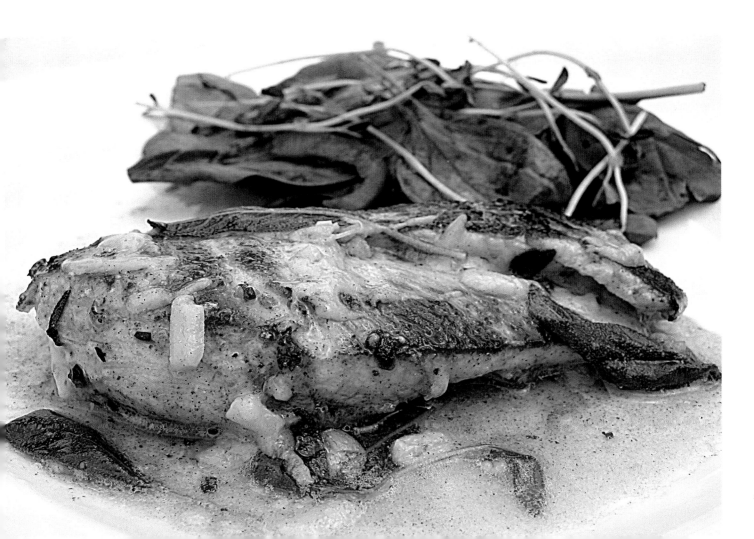

KAFFIR LIME PORK STIR-FRY

1 Tbsp ginger, finely grated
6 kaffir lime leaves, shredded
1 small red chilli, deseeded, sliced thinly
2 1/2 Tbsp brown sugar
2 Tbsp (40ml) lime juice
1/3 cup (85ml) gluten free soy sauce
3 Tbsp sesame oil
600g lean pork, cut into strips
250g dried rice noodles
boiling water
1 bunch (110g) bok choy, rinsed
1 1/4 cups (125g) snow peas, trimmed
150g broccoli florettes
1/4 cup fresh coriander, roughly chopped

Combine ginger, lime leaves, chilli, brown sugar, lime juice, 1 tablespoon soy sauce and 1 tablespoon oil in a bowl. Add pork strips, toss well to combine. Cover, refrigerate for 3 to 4 hours, or overnight.

Soak noodles in a large bowl of boiled water for 5 minutes (or until tender). Drain and set aside.

Heat remaining oil in a wok, stir-fry pork until just cooked. Add bok choy, snow peas, broccoli and remaining soy sauce. Stir-fry until vegetables just tender. Add noodles, stir-fry to combine. Sprinkle with coriander before serving.

Serves 4

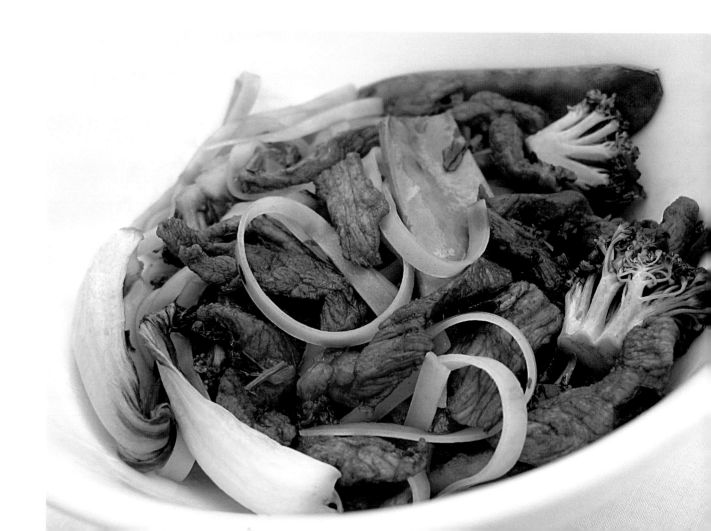

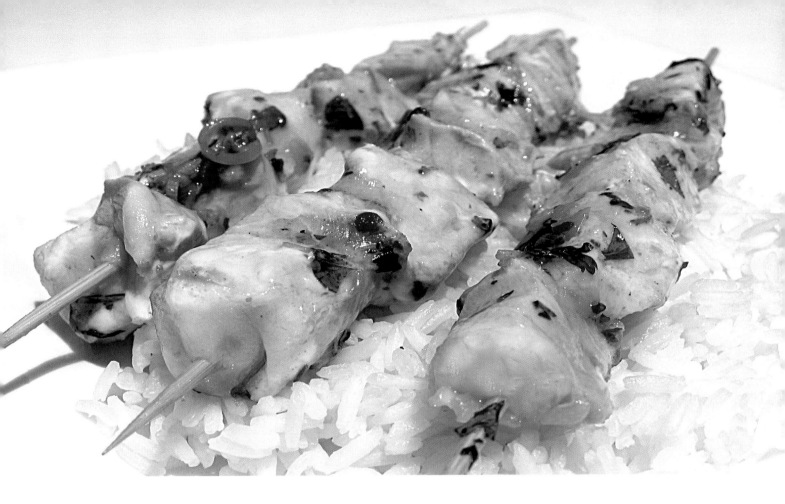

FRAGRANT SNAPPER KEBABS WITH JASMINE RICE

12 wooden skewers
1/2 cup fresh coriander, chopped
2 tsp fresh ginger, grated
3 cloves garlic, crushed
2 tsp lemon grass, sliced
1 small chilli, deseeded, finely chopped
2 Tbsp sesame oil
6 x 250g snapper fillets, cut into 2cm cubes
2 cups (440g) jasmine rice, cooked

Pre-heat oven to 180°C. Grease two baking trays. Soak wooden skewers in water for 10 minutes.

In a small mixing bowl, combine coriander, ginger, garlic, lemon grass, chilli and sesame oil. Add snapper pieces to bowl of marinade, toss gently to coat. Thread snapper pieces onto skewers. Place skewers on baking trays, bake in pre-heated oven for 10 minutes. Serve on top of cooked jasmine rice.

Serves 4

SPICY LENTILS

1 cup (200g) red lentils
1 Tbsp olive oil
4 medium (560g) tomatoes, chopped
2 medium (240g) carrots, diced
1 small (100g) zucchini, grated
3 cloves garlic, crushed
2 tsp ground cumin
2 tsp ground coriander
1 tsp paprika
2 tsp ground turmeric
1 tsp brown sugar
1/2 cup fresh parsley, finely chopped
salt, freshly ground black pepper to taste

Add lentils to a large saucepan of boiling water. Reduce heat to low, simmer, uncovered, for 8 to 10 minutes or until the lentils are just tender. Drain.

Heat olive oil in a large frying pan over medium-low heat and sauté tomatoes, carrot, zucchini, garlic, cumin, coriander, paprika, turmeric and sugar. Cook, simmering for approximately 10 minutes. Stir in lentils, parsley, salt and pepper. Heat through and serve.

Serves 4

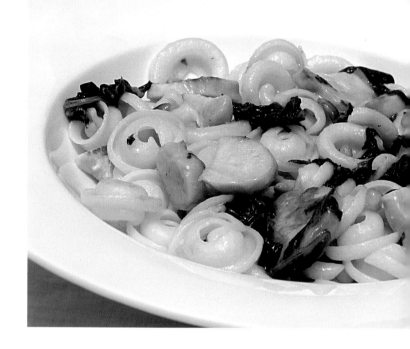

SMOKED CHICKEN PASTA

500g gluten free pasta
1/4 cup (65ml) olive oil
2 cloves garlic, crushed
1 large fillet (200g) smoked chicken, sliced
2 cups (70g) baby spinach leaves
1/3 cup (55g) pine nuts
1/2 cup (60g) parmesan cheese, grated
salt, freshly ground black pepper to taste

Cook gluten free pasta in a large pot of boiling water until just tender. Drain and return to the saucepan. Stir through 2 tablespoons of olive oil, cover to keep warm.

In a large frying pan, sauté garlic, smoked chicken, spinach and pine nuts in remaining olive oil until chicken and pine nuts are golden brown and spinach has wilted. Add cooked gluten free pasta and parmesan cheese to pan, toss through over medium heat until cheese melted. Add salt and pepper to taste, and additional olive oil if desired.

Serves 4

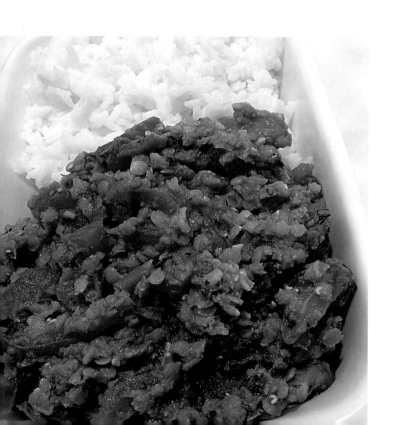

BARBECUED PESTO STEAK WITH POTATO WEDGES

8 new potatoes (720g), washed, skin remaining
2 Tbsp gluten free cornflour
1 tsp gluten free chicken stock powder
1/2 tsp salt
2 Tbsp olive oil
4 x 200g T-bone steaks
8 Tbsp gluten free prepared pesto sauce (see p. 22)

Pre-heat oven to 200°C. Cut potatoes in half. Cut each half into 11/2cm-thick wedges.
In a plastic bag, combine cornflour, chicken stock powder and salt. Toss potato wedges in seasoned flour, shake excess. Potatoes should only be lightly coated. Place coated wedges in a single layer on a baking tray lined with greaseproof paper. Brush with olive oil. Cook in pre-heated oven for 10 minutes. Reduce oven temperature to 180°C, and continue to bake, turning after 10 minutes, for further 20 minutes or until crisp and golden brown.

Cook steaks to liking on barbecue or chargrill. Top steaks with 1 tablespoon of prepared pesto sauce, with wedges and another tablespoon of pesto on the side.

Serves 4

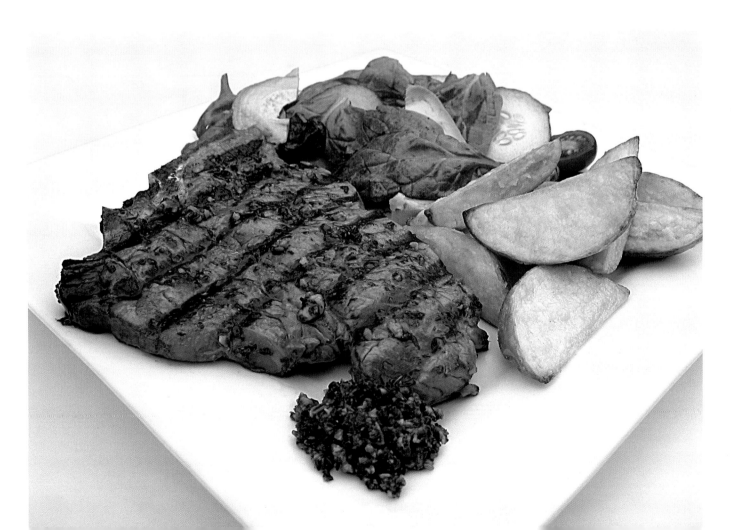

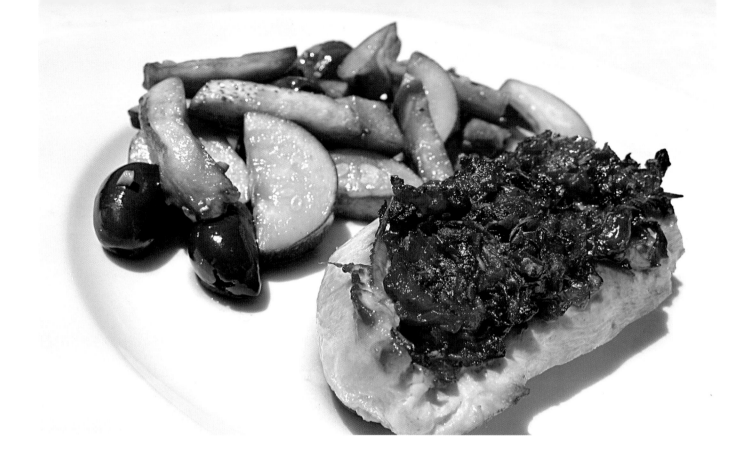

CHICKEN WITH OLIVE, SUN-DRIED TOMATO AND BASIL SERVED WITH MEDITERRANEAN VEGETABLES

2 Tbsp (30g) black olives, pitted
1/2 cup (80g) sun-dried tomatoes
1/2 cup fresh basil leaves
1 Tbsp olive oil
salt, freshly ground black pepper to taste
4 x 200g chicken breasts
1 Tbsp olive oil, extra

Pre-heat oven to 170°C.

In a small bowl, combine olives, sun-dried tomatoes, basil, oil, salt and pepper. Purée with hand-held blender (or crush with mortar and pestle) until mixture smooth and even.

In a large frying pan, pan-fry chicken fillets in extra olive oil over medium-low heat until lightly browned but cooked through. Remove from heat and place on baking tray. Spread topping evenly over four chicken breasts. Cover baking tray with foil. Place in oven and bake for 10 to 15 minutes. Serve with Mediterranean vegetables on the side.

Mediterranean vegetables
1 Tbsp olive oil
2 cloves garlic, crushed
2 medium (300g) zucchini, cut in half, sliced
1 medium (330g) eggplant, cut into strips
1/2 cup (70g) Kalamata olives, whole
2 Tbsp balsamic vinegar
1/2 cup (125ml) gluten free vegetable stock

Heat olive oil in large frying pan over medium heat. Sauté garlic until slightly browned. Add all other vegetables, balsamic vinegar and vegetable stock. Simmer for 3 to 5 minutes, stirring occasionally until stock almost evaporated and vegetables are tender.

Serves 4

SMOKED TUNA RISOTTO

1 Tbsp olive oil
1 tsp saffron threads
2 1/2 cups (550g) Arborio rice
1/2 cup (125ml) white wine
8 cups (2L) gluten free vegetable stock
400g tinned smoked tuna in oil, drained
1 cup (160g) frozen peas
2 medium (400g) zucchini, cut in half, sliced
1/2 cup (60g) parmesan cheese, grated
1/4 cup fresh parsley, chopped
salt, freshly ground black pepper to taste

Heat olive oil in a large saucepan. Add saffron and stir over medium heat for 2 minutes. Add rice and stir for 1 to 2 minutes or until rice is well coated with oil and saffron mixture.
Heat vegetable stock in medium-sized saucepan. Keep covered, simmering over low heat. Add wine to rice and stir until absorbed. Add 1 cup of heated stock, continue stirring through rice until it is all absorbed. Repeat this process, adding 1/2 cup of stock at a time, until all but last 1/2 cup of stock is used. Add smoked tuna, peas, zucchini pieces, parmesan cheese and parsley. Stir until well combined. Add last 1/2 cup of stock, stirring until all absorbed and rice tender. Taste, season with salt and pepper.

Serves 6

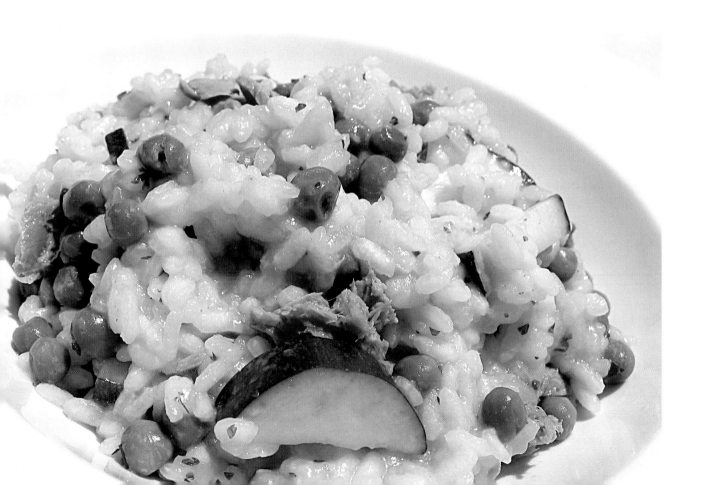

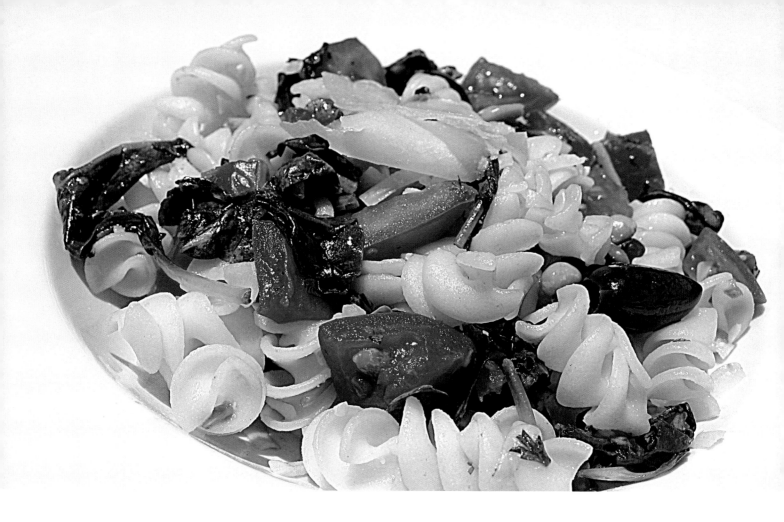

FRESH MEDITERRANEAN PASTA WITH PECORINO CHEESE

500g gluten free pasta
2 Tbsp olive oil
1/2 cup (80g) pine nuts
4 cups (130g) baby spinach leaves
1 cup (140g) Kalamata olives, pitted
6 medium (480g) Roma tomatoes, chopped
4 Tbsp fresh basil, chopped
2 Tbsp fresh parsley, chopped
2/3 cup (70g) pecorino cheese, crumbled
salt, freshly ground black pepper to taste
shaved pecorino cheese, extra

Cook gluten free pasta in a large saucepan of boiling water, until just tender. Drain, return to the saucepan, stir through 1 tablespoon of olive oil and cover to keep warm.

In a large heavy-based pan, heat remaining olive oil over medium heat. Add pine nuts, toss until golden brown. Add spinach leaves, olives, tomatoes, basil and parsley, cook until spinach has wilted. Finally, add cheese to pan, heat until warmed through and slightly melted. Season with salt and pepper to taste. Toss sauce through the cooked gluten free pasta.

Serves 4

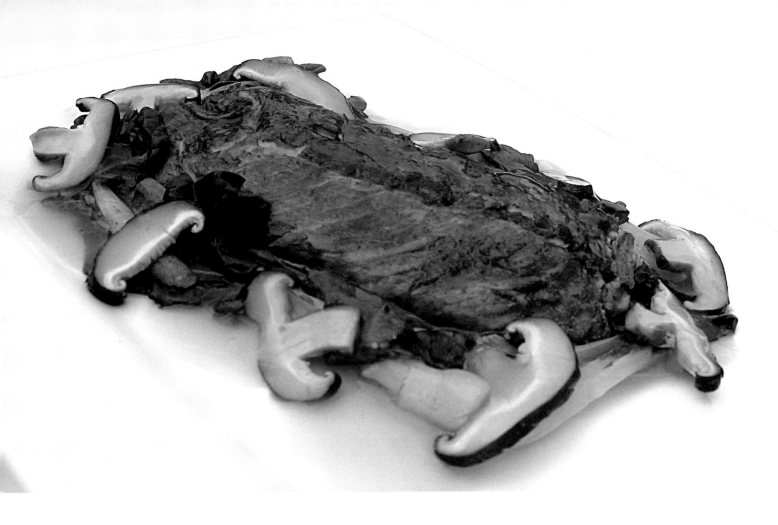

SOY AND GINGER BARRAMUNDI

3 Tbsp gluten free soy sauce
3 Tbsp fresh ginger, grated
2 tsp sesame oil
2 tsp lemon juice
2 Tbsp gluten free cornflour
4 x 250g fillets barramundi
1 cup (250ml) gluten free vegetable stock
2 tsp gluten free cornflour
1 tsp sesame oil, extra
2 bunches (220g) baby bok choy, rinsed and trimmed
8 shitake mushrooms, sliced

Combine soy sauce, ginger, sesame oil, lemon juice and cornflour in a large bowl. Place barramundi fillets in bowl, toss lightly in marinade, ensuring fillets coated. Cover, place in refrigerator for 2 to 3 hours or overnight

Place marinated barramundi fillets in a single layer in a bamboo steamer (see hint), set above a saucepan of boiling water. Retain remaining marinade. Steam for 8 to 10 minutes.

In a small bowl, combine remaining marinade, vegetable stock and cornflour together. Mix well to ensure smooth consistency. Heat extra sesame oil in frying pan over medium-high heat. Add bok choy and mushrooms. Sauté for 1 to 2 minutes. Add vegetable stock, heat for further 2 to 3 minutes or until sauce has thickened. Place steamed barramundi on plate, serve with stir-fried bok choy and mushroom sauce.

Hint: If you do not own a steamer, barramundi fillets can be baked in an oven. Place each fillet on a piece of foil sprayed with cooking spray. Wrap and bake in moderate oven for 12 minutes or according to liking.

Serves 4

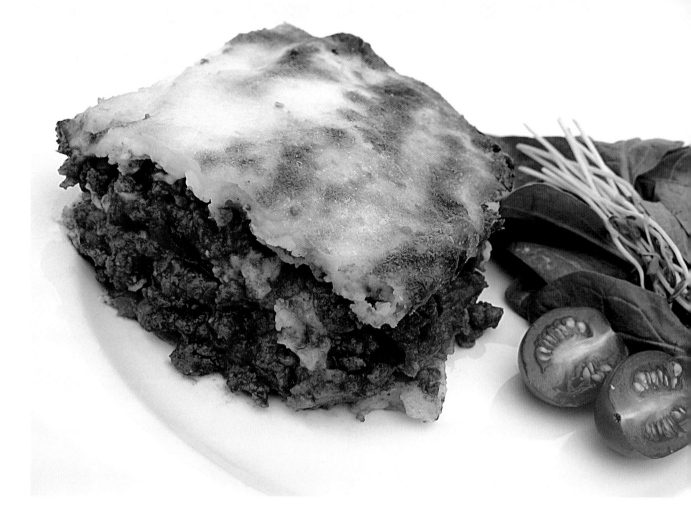

LASAGNE

1 Tbsp olive oil
1kg lean beef mince
300g lean bacon, diced
2 cloves garlic, crushed
2 tsp cayenne pepper
1/2 tsp chilli powder (optional)
salt, freshly ground black pepper to taste
2 3/4 cups (700ml) tomato purée
180g mushrooms, sliced
1 medium (140g) carrot, grated
4 cups (1L) reduced fat milk •
3 Tbsp gluten free cornflour
3 cups (300g) reduced fat tasty cheese, grated
1 x packet gluten free lasagne sheets

Pre-heat oven to 180°C. In a large heavy-based frying pan, heat olive oil over medium heat. Add beef mince, bacon and garlic. Sauté until beef browned. Add herbs and spices, tomato purée, mushrooms and carrot. Simmer over medium heat for 10 minutes, stirring occasionally.

In a small mixing bowl, combine 1/4 cup milk with cornflour to form a paste. Add remaining milk, mixing well to ensure evenly combined. Pour into a saucepan, stirring continually over medium heat until thickened. Do not boil. Add grated cheese, stir until melted.

Run lasagne sheets under cold water or prepare as per packet directions. Place a layer of prepared lasagne sheets on bottom of lasagne dish. Spread half of the meat mixture evenly over lasagne sheets. Top with 1/3 of the cheese sauce. Top this with another layer of lasagne sheets, then remaining meat sauce, then 1/3 cheese sauce. Finally, top with final layer of lasagne sheets and remaining cheese sauce. Bake in pre-heated oven for 20 minutes or until golden brown.

Serves 8   • See recipe hints p.132

ASIAN DUCK AND PEA RISOTTO

6 x 180g duck maryland pieces
1/2 cup (125ml) gluten free soy sauce
2 cloves garlic, crushed
2 tsp ginger, grated
2 Tbsp sesame oil
salt, freshly ground black pepper to taste
1 cup (250ml) boiling water
1 cup (40g) dried shitake mushrooms
8 cups (2L) gluten free chicken stock
2 sticks (180g) celery, sliced
1 Tbsp sesame oil, extra
2 1/2 cups (550g) Arborio rice
1 cup (160g) frozen peas

In a large bowl, combine soy sauce, garlic, ginger, sesame oil, salt and pepper. Add whole maryland pieces, toss to coat well. Cover, then refrigerate for 3 to 4 hours or overnight.

Pre-heat oven to 180°C. Place marinated duck marylands in a baking dish and bake in pre-heated oven for 20 to 25 minutes or until cooked. In a heat-proof bowl, pour boiling water over dried shitake mushrooms. Leave to soak for 30 minutes. Heat chicken stock in medium saucepan. Leave simmering, covered, over medium-low heat. In a large stockpot, sauté celery in sesame oil until tender and slightly browned. Add rice, stir through celery and oil. Add mushrooms and water used for soaking and remaining marinade juices. Stir constantly over medium heat. Add 1/2 cup of hot chicken stock, stirring through rice mixture. Continue stirring until all liquid absorbed. Repeat this process with additions of 1/2 cup of warm chicken stock, until rice is tender. When adding the last of the chicken stock, also stir through peas and salt and pepper to taste. Serve risotto in the centre of the plate, top with roasted duck.

Serves 6

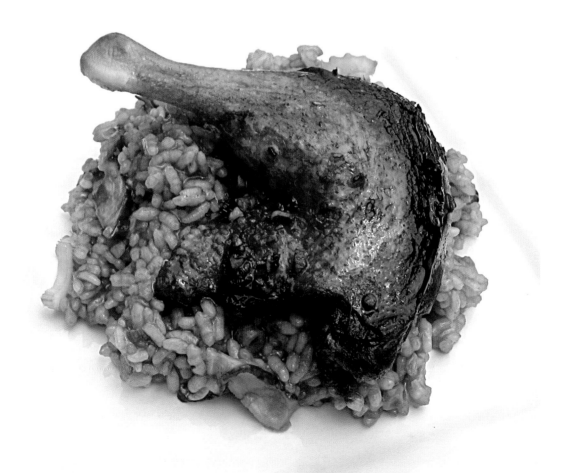

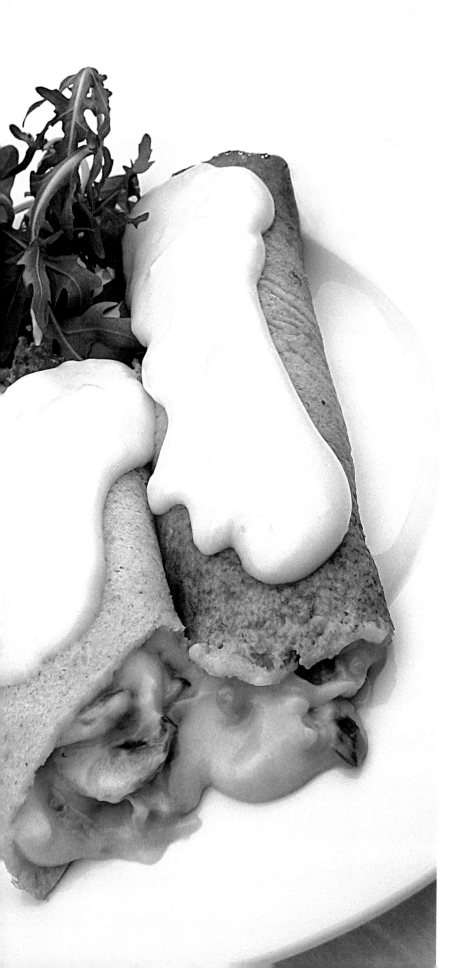

MUSHROOM AND HAM CREPES

Crepes
3/4 cup (130g) rice flour
1/2 cup (75g) gluten free cornflour
1/3 cup (30g) soy flour •
3/4 tsp bicarb soda
2 eggs, lightly beaten
11/2 cups (375ml) reduced fat milk •
2 Tbsp butter, melted

Cheese Sauce
2 cups (500ml) reduced fat milk •
2 Tbsp gluten free cornflour
2 cups (200g) reduced fat tasty cheese, grated
salt, freshly ground black pepper to taste

Filling
15 (300g) mushrooms, sliced
200g gluten free Virginian ham, shredded

Crepes: Sift flours and bicarb soda three times into a bowl. Make a well in the middle, add beaten eggs and milk and blend forming smooth batter. Stir in melted butter. Cover with plastic wrap, set aside for 20 minutes.

Heat a heavy-based fryng pan over medium heat, spray with cooking spray. Pour batter into warmed frying pan. Turn when bubbles appear over crepe. Cook other side, repeat to make eight crepes. Set crepes aside, keeping warm.

Cheese Sauce: In a small mixing bowl, combine 1/4 cup milk with cornflour to form a paste. Add remaining milk, mix well to ensure evenly combined. Pour into a saucepan, stirring constantly over medium heat until thickened. Do not boil. Add grated cheese, salt and pepper. Stir until cheese melted.

Filling: In a heavy based frying pan, sauté mushrooms and ham until lightly browned. Add mushroom and ham mixture to half of the cheese sauce. Place spoonfuls of this mixture across the centre of each cooked crepe. Roll up and top with remaining cheese sauce.

Serves 4   • • See recipe hints p.132

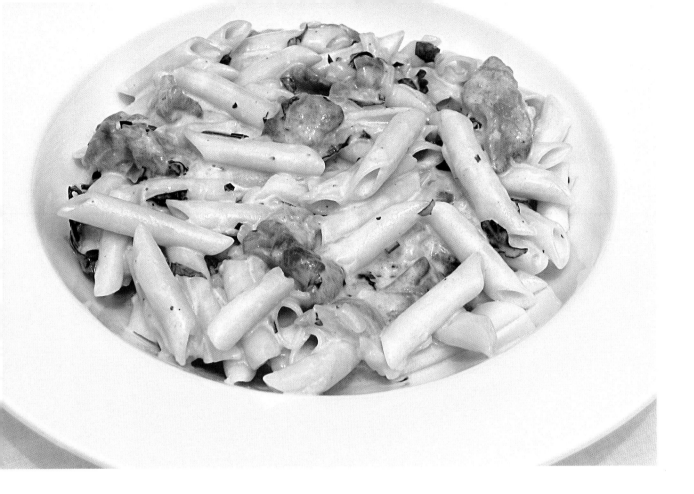

SMOKED SALMON PASTA

500g gluten free pasta
2 cups (500ml) reduced fat cream
1/2 cup (125ml) dry white wine
1 clove garlic, crushed
3/4 cup (90g) parmesan cheese, grated
1/3 cup fresh continental parsley, chopped
1 tsp ground black pepper
1 tsp lemon rind, finely grated
200g smoked salmon, cut into thin strips
salt, freshly ground black pepper to taste

Cook gluten free pasta in a large saucepan of boiling water, until just tender. Drain, return to the saucepan and cover to keep warm.

Place the cream, wine and garlic in a large frying pan and heat over high heat, for 1 minute, stirring constantly. Reduce heat to medium and simmer, uncovered, stirring occasionally, for 5 to 6 minutes or until the sauce thickens slightly. Remove from the heat. Stir in cheese, parsley, pepper and lemon rind, stirring until cheese melted. Pour sauce and smoked salmon into the saucepan with the cooked gluten free pasta and toss to combine. Taste, season with additional salt and pepper as desired.

Serves 4

SEEDED MUSTARD BEEF RISOTTO

400g lean sirloin steak, cut into strips
2 tsp olive oil
12 (250g) mushrooms, sliced
9 cups (2250ml) gluten free beef stock
2 1/2 cups (550g) Arborio rice
3/4 cup (90g) parmesan cheese, grated
4 Tbsp gluten free seeded wholegrain mustard
2 Tbsp fresh parsley, chopped

Sauté beef strips in olive oil in large frying pan over medium heat until lightly browned. Add sliced mushrooms, sauté until tender. Set aside.

Heat beef stock in medium-sized saucepan, keep covered, simmering over low heat. Into a large stockpot, pour 1 cup of heated beef stock. Add rice, stir until nearly all the stock is absorbed. Add another 1/2 cup of heated stock. Continue stirring through rice until absorbed. Repeat this process until all but last 1/2 cup of stock used. Stir through beef, mushrooms, parmesan cheese, mustard and parsley. Add final 1/2 cup of beef stock, stir until all liquid absorbed and rice is tender.

If desired, serve with mustard pouring sauce: combine 1 Tbsp gluten free seeded mustard, 1 cup gluten free beef stock and 1 Tbsp maize cornflour. Heat, stirring until thickened. Drizzle over top of risotto.

Serves 4-6

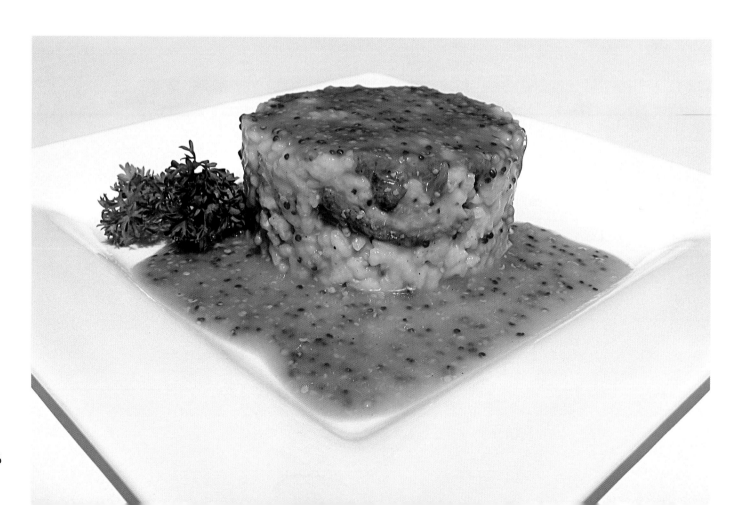

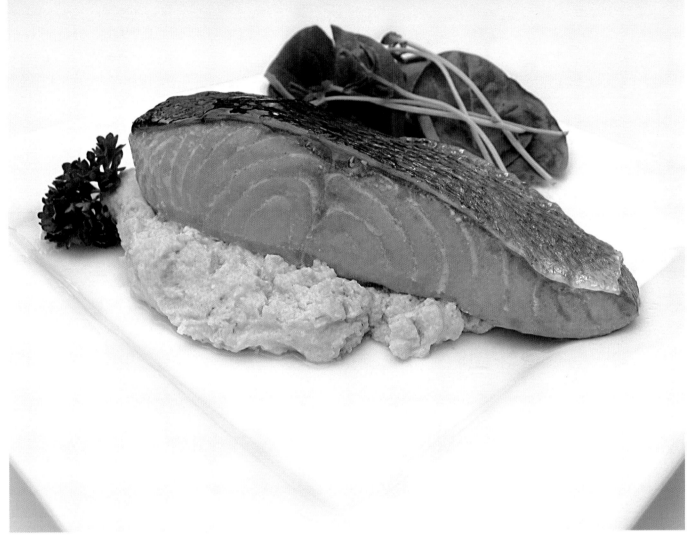

BAKED ATLANTIC SALMON ON SOFT BLUE CHEESE POLENTA

4 x 180g Atlantic salmon fillets
olive oil
3 cups (750ml) reduced fat milk •
2 cloves garlic, crushed
2/3 cup (135g) instant polenta
salt, freshly ground black pepper to taste
80g strong blue cheese, approx.

Pre-heat oven to 180°C. Place serving plates into oven. Also place salmon fillets on greased oven tray, brush with olive oil, and bake for approximately 10 to 12 minutes or to liking.

While salmon is cooking, heat milk and garlic in a medium-sized saucepan until almost boiling. Add polenta, and stir until the mixture boils. Reduce heat to low, stir constantly for further 3 to 5 minutes until the polenta is cooked. Polenta should be texture of smooth mashed potato. Stir through blue cheese, adjusting amount according to taste preference. Season with salt and pepper. Serve soft polenta on warmed plates, top with baked salmon fillets.

Serves 4   • See recipe hints p.132

EASY CHICKEN STIR-FRY

2 Tbsp sesame oil
600g chicken breast fillets, cut into strips
1 small red chilli, seeded and finely chopped, or $1/2$ tsp chilli powder (optional)
1 bunch (110g) bok choy, trimmed
1 1$1/4$ cups (125g) snow peas, trimmed
250g mushrooms, sliced
200g baby corn pieces
1 Tbsp gluten free cornflour
2 Tbsp gluten free soy sauce
1 cup (250ml) gluten free chicken stock

Heat sesame oil in a wok over medium heat. Add chicken and chilli. Stir-fry for 4 to 5 minutes or until chicken is browned. Turn heat up to medium-high. Add vegetables, stir-fry for further 2 to 3 minutes or until vegetables are tender.

In a small bowl, mix cornflour together with soy sauce and a little chicken stock to form a paste. Gradually add remaining liquid chicken stock, stir until well blended. Pour over chicken and vegetables, heat through until thickened. Serve on rice or rice noodles.

Serves 4

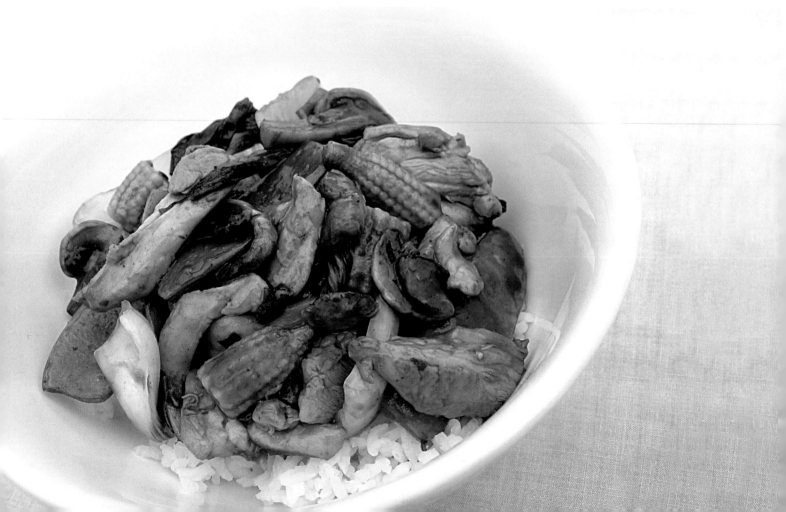

SPAGHETTI BOLOGNAISE

1 Tbsp olive oil
800g lean minced beef
10 (200g) rashers rindless bacon, diced
2 cloves garlic, crushed
2 2/3 cups (700ml) tomato purée
200g mushrooms, sliced
2 tsp cayenne pepper
1/2 tsp chilli powder (optional)
salt, freshly ground black pepper to taste
1 x 500g packet gluten free spaghetti, cooked
parmesan cheese, if desired

In a large heavy-based frying pan, heat olive oil over medium heat. Add beef mince, bacon and garlic. Sauté until beef is browned, breaking up any lumps of mince. Add tomato purée, mushrooms, cayenne and chilli. Simmer over medium heat for 10 minutes, stirring occasionally. Taste, season with salt and pepper. Spoon over warm, cooked, gluten free spaghetti. Serve with grated parmesan cheese as desired.

Serves 4

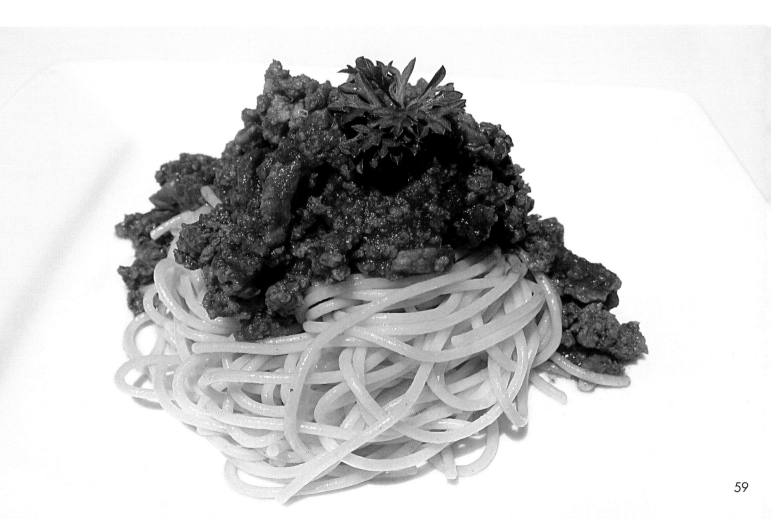

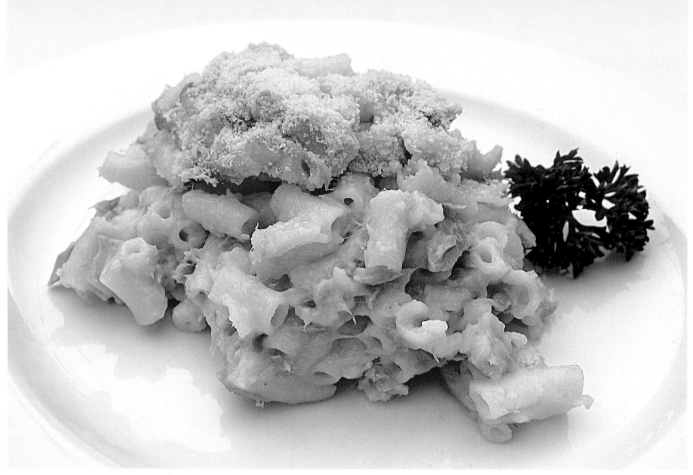

TUNA MACARONI CHEESE BAKE

250g gluten free macaroni
1/3 cup (40g) gluten free breadcrumbs
1/3 cup (40g) parmesan cheese, grated
2 1/4 cups (560ml) reduced fat milk •
4 Tbsp (50g) gluten free cornflour
425g canned tuna, drained
2 cups (200g) reduced fat tasty cheese, grated
salt, freshly ground black pepper to taste

Pre-heat oven to 180°C. Cook gluten free pasta in a large saucepan of boiling water, until just tender. Drain, set aside.

In a small mixing bowl, combine breadcrumbs and parmesan cheese. Set aside.

In a small mixing bowl, combine 1/4 cup milk with cornflour to form a paste. Add remaining milk, mixing well to ensure evenly combined. Pour into a saucepan, stirring constantly over medium heat until thickened. Do not boil. Add tuna, grated cheese, salt and pepper, stirring until cheese has melted. Pour over cooked pasta, mix through until well combined. Pour into greased baking tray, and top with combined cheese and breadcrumb topping. Bake in pre-heated oven for 15 to 20 minutes or until golden brown.

Serves 6-8   • See recipe hints p.132

PORK & CANNELLINI CASSEROLE

1/4 cup (35g) gluten free cornflour
salt, freshly ground black pepper
1200g lean pork, diced
1 Tbsp olive oil
2 cloves garlic, crushed
1 x 425g canned tomatoes, crushed
1/2 cup (125ml) tomato purée
2 small onions, whole (peeled)
1 1/2 cups (375ml) gluten free beef stock
1 small fresh rosemary sprig
4 cups (135g) baby spinach leaves
6 medium (120g) mushrooms, cut into quarters
1 x 400g can cannellini beans

In a shallow bowl, mix cornflour, salt and pepper.
Dust diced pork in seasoned flour. Heat olive oil
in large non-stick stockpot. Add half of the pork
pieces, cook, tossing for 2 to 3 minutes or until
golden brown. Set browned pork aside on plate,
cover to keep warm. Repeat for remaining pork.

Add garlic to pan, sauté lightly in meat juices.
Add tomatoes, tomato purée, whole onions, beef
stock, rosemary and cooked pork pieces to pan.
Stir, and bring to the boil over medium heat.
Reduce heat to very low, cook covered, stirring
occasionally, for 60 minutes or until pork very
tender. Remove from heat, and remove onions.
Stir in baby spinach leaves, mushrooms and
canned beans. Taste, season with salt and
pepper as desired. Let stand for 5 minutes or
until mushrooms softened.

Serves 4

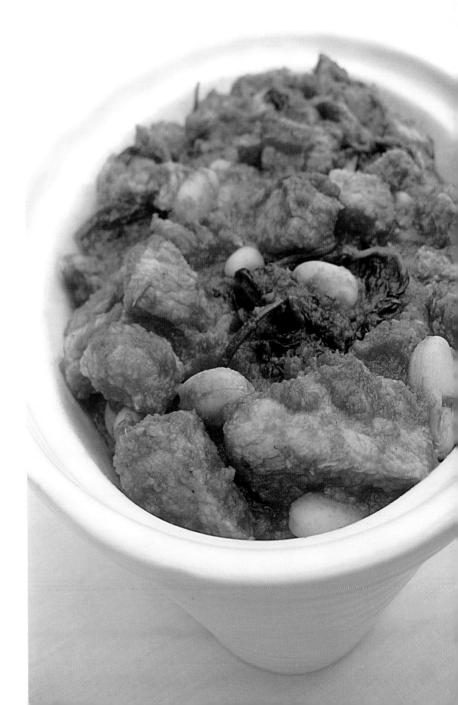

BEEF KOFTA

12 wooden skewers
600g lean minced beef
2 eggs, lightly beaten
1/3 cup (40g) gluten free breadcrumbs
1/4 cup fresh parsley, chopped
1 tsp ground cinnamon
11/2 Tbsp ground cumin
1/2 tsp chilli powder (more to taste)
3 tsp ground turmeric
11/2 tsp ground allspice

Tahini sauce
1/2 cup (125ml) gluten free natural yoghurt
2 tsp lemon juice
2 Tbsp tahini (sesame paste)
1 clove garlic, crushed

Soak wooden skewers in water. Add beef mince, eggs, breadcrumbs, parsley and spices into a large mixing bowl. Mix with hands until well combined. Shape 1/4 cup of beef mixture around a wooden skewer. Repeat for remaining beef mixture. Cook kofta under grill or pan-fry until browned all over and cooked through. Serve with Tahini sauce.

Tahini sauce: Combine ingredients in small jar, shake well to combine.

Serves 4-6

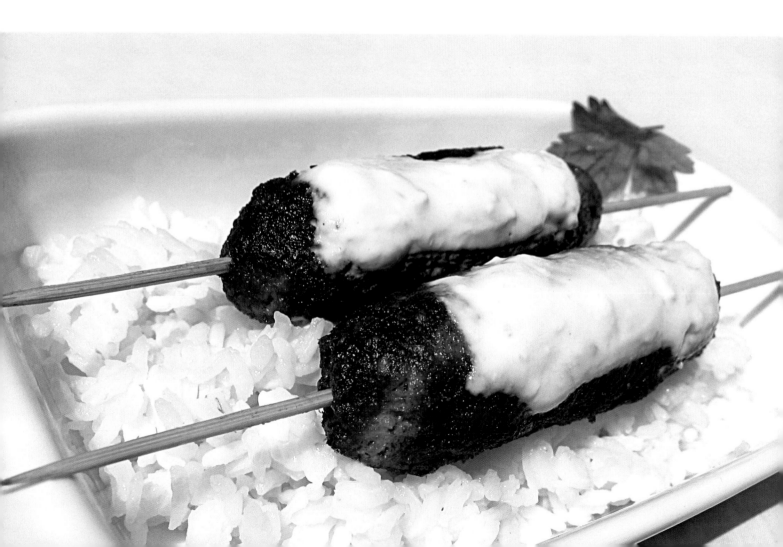

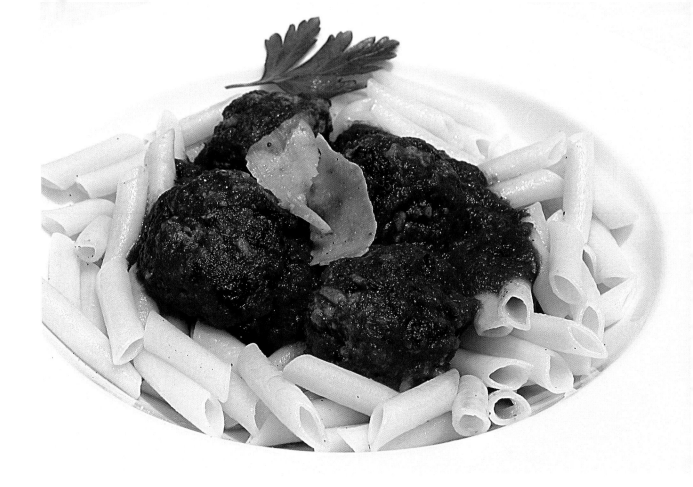

PENNE WITH MEATBALLS

1kg lean minced beef
1 cup (220g) cooked long grain rice
3/4 cup (90g) parmesan cheese, grated
1 egg, beaten
2 cloves garlic, crushed
4 Tbsp fresh basil, chopped
1/4 cup fresh parsley, chopped
1/2 tsp cayenne pepper
salt, freshly ground black pepper to taste
2 cups (500ml) puréed tomato
1/4 cup fresh basil, chopped, extra
500g gluten free penne pasta, cooked
additional parmesan cheese, if desired

Combine mince, cooked rice, cheese, egg, garlic, basil, parsley, cayenne, salt and pepper in a large mixing bowl. Shape into golf ball-size balls and cook in a large non-stick frying pan over medium heat until browned and cooked through. Pour puréed tomato over meatballs, add extra basil. Cook, simmering for 2 to 3 minutes. Spoon meatballs and sauce over cooked pasta, top with parmesan cheese if desired.

Serves 4

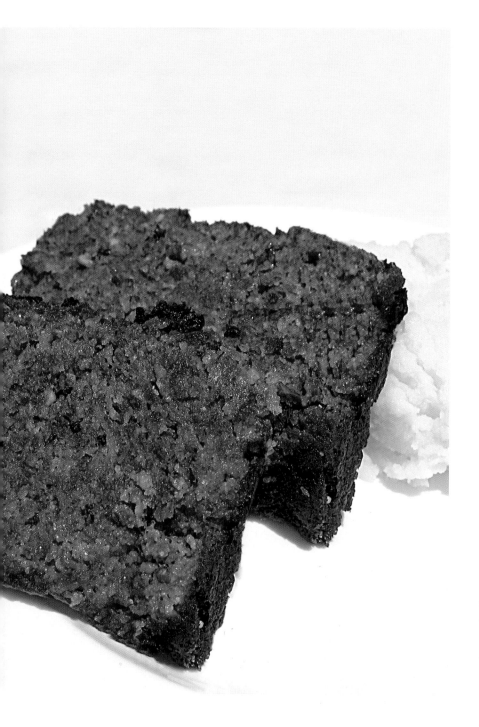

SPANISH MEATLOAF WITH GARLIC MASH

750g lean minced beef
1/2 cup (125ml) tomato paste
3/4 cup (90g) gluten free breadcrumbs
2 eggs, lightly beaten
2 cloves garlic, crushed
1/2 cup fresh parsley, chopped
3/4 tsp ground ginger
1 tsp chilli powder (optional)
1 1/2 tsp cayenne pepper
1 1/2 tsp sweet paprika
salt, freshly ground black pepper to taste
non-stick cooking spray

Garlic Mash
4 large (720g) potatoes, peeled and quartered
2 cloves garlic, crushed
2 Tbsp butter
1/3 cup (85ml) reduced fat milk
salt, freshly ground black pepper to taste

Pre-heat oven to 180°C. Line 22cm rectangular loaf pan with foil, and spray with non-stick cooking spray.

Combine all ingredients in a large bowl. Mix well, using your hands. Press into prepared loaf pan and bake in pre-heated oven for 40 to 45 minutes or until cooked through. Let meatloaf stand for 5 minutes before removing from pan and slicing. Serve on top of garlic mash.

Garlic Mash: Cook potatoes in pot of boiling water until soft. Drain, place in bowl of food processor. Turn food processor to high setting, add crushed garlic, butter, milk, salt and pepper to taste. Blend until smooth and even in consistency. Add more milk if required.

Serves 4

CHICKEN FRIED RICE

2 cups (440g) long grain rice
1 Tbsp sesame oil
1 1/2 tsp Chinese five spice powder
1 1/2 Tbsp fresh coriander, chopped
1/2 tsp ground cumin
1 clove garlic, crushed
1 Tbsp ginger, grated
500g chicken breast, sliced
1 medium (140g) carrot, sliced into matchstick pieces
1/2 cup (80g) frozen peas
1/4 (75g) green capsicum, thinly sliced into 2cm lengths
1/4 (75g) red capsicum, thinly sliced into 2cm lengths
1/2 cup (60g) bamboo shoots
1 cup (50g) bean sprouts
2 eggs, lightly beaten
1/4 cup (65ml) gluten free soy sauce
2 Tbsp sesame oil, extra
salt, freshly ground pepper to taste

Cook rice in boiling water until just tender. Drain, set aside.

In large frying pan heat oil, spices, garlic and ginger over medium heat. Add sliced chicken breast, heat through until just cooked. Add carrot, peas, capsicum, bean shoots and bean sprouts. Make a well in the centre of frying pan and add beaten eggs, stir until just cooked, breaking up egg as cooking. Continue to heat until capsicum and carrot are tender. Finally, add rice, soy sauce and extra sesame oil. Stir though until well combined. Taste, season with salt and pepper.

Serves 4

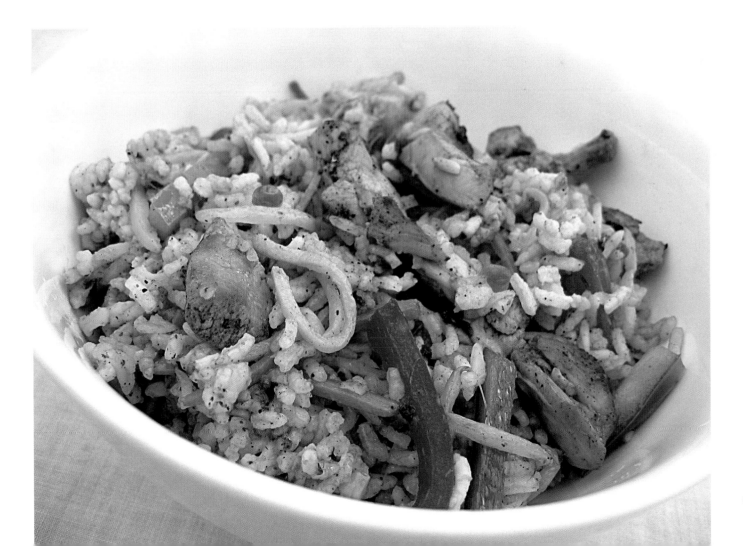

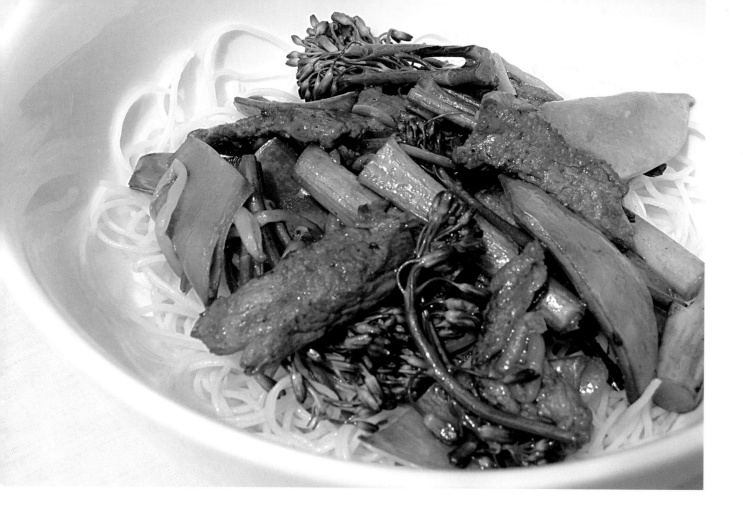

EASY BEEF STIR-FRY

400g beef rump steak
2 Tbsp sesame oil
2 cloves garlic, crushed
3 tsp fresh ginger, grated
1 Tbsp gluten free oyster sauce
1 Tbsp gluten free cornflour
1/4 tsp chilli powder
1 cup (250ml) gluten free beef stock
1 Tbsp sesame oil, extra
1 bunch (260g) broccolini, cut into 3cm lengths
2 cups (200g) snow peas, trimmed
1 cup (50g) bean sprouts, rinsed

Slice beef into very thin slices. Combine oil, garlic and ginger in a bowl. Add beef strips, toss to ensure well coated. Refrigerate for 2 to 3 hours.

In a small bowl, combine oyster sauce with cornflour and chilli powder to form a paste. Add beef stock slowly, stirring well until evenly blended.

Heat extra oil in a wok over medium-high heat. Add beef, cook 2 minutes, or until lightly browned. Add vegetables; stir-fry for 2 to 4 minutes or until tender. Pour in prepared sauce, heat through for 1 to 2 minutes or until thickened slightly and coating all meat and vegetables. Serve immediately over steamed rice or rice noodles.

Serves 4

SEAFOOD PASTA WITH SALSA VERDE

1 x 500g packet gluten free pasta
1/2 cup prepared salsa verde (see p. 22)
1 Tbsp olive oil
2 medium (250g) calamari hoods (squid tube), sliced into rings
250g firm white fish fillets, cubed
500g green prawns, shelled, de-veined
2 cloves garlic, crushed
500g mussel meat
1/2 cup (125ml) reduced fat cream
2 Tbsp dry white wine
salt, freshly ground black pepper to taste

Cook gluten free pasta in a large pot of boiling water until just tender. Drain and return to saucepan. Stir through salsa verde until evenly combined. Cover saucepan to keep pasta warm.

While pasta is cooking, heat oil in large frying pan. Sauté calamari, fish, prawns and garlic for 2 minutes, tossing gently. Add mussels, cream and wine. Stir though to ensure well combined. Reduce heat to low, simmer for 3 to 4 minutes. Taste, season with salt and pepper. Spoon prepared pasta over four bowls and top with seafood sauce.

Serves 4

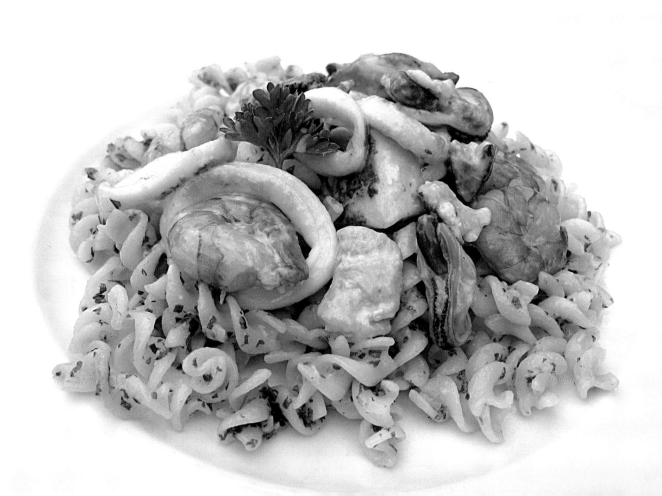

BASIL AND MOZZARELLA STUFFED CHICKEN PARCELS

5 large (750g) chicken thigh fillets
2/3 cup (80g) gluten free breadcrumbs
1 egg
3 Tbsp gluten free prepared pesto paste (see p. 22)
80g mozzarella cheese, 8 x (2cm x 1cm) pieces
8 medium basil leaves
8 slices (100g) prosciutto

Garlic cream sauce
1/4 cup (65ml) reduced fat cream
1 clove garlic, crushed
salt, freshly ground pepper to taste

Heat oven to 180°C. In a food processor, combine chicken fillets, breadcrumbs, egg and pesto. Blend until just combined, do not over-process. Portion out the chicken mince mixture into eight evenly sized balls.

Flatten each ball, and place a piece of mozzarella cheese and a basil leaf in the middle. Re-form ball around cheese and basil, ensuring cheese is fully encased within chicken mixture. Shape into parcels, approximately 3cm wide in diameter and 5cm long. Wrap each chicken parcel in a slice of prosciutto and secure with a toothpick. Place chicken parcels on a greased baking tray. Bake in pre-heated oven for 20 minutes. Remove chicken parcels from oven. Drizzle a little prepared garlic cream sauce over chicken prior to serving.

Garlic cream sauce: In a small saucepan, heat cream and garlic, adding salt and pepper to taste. Simmer for 3 to 5 minutes, or until sauce thickened slightly.

Serves 4

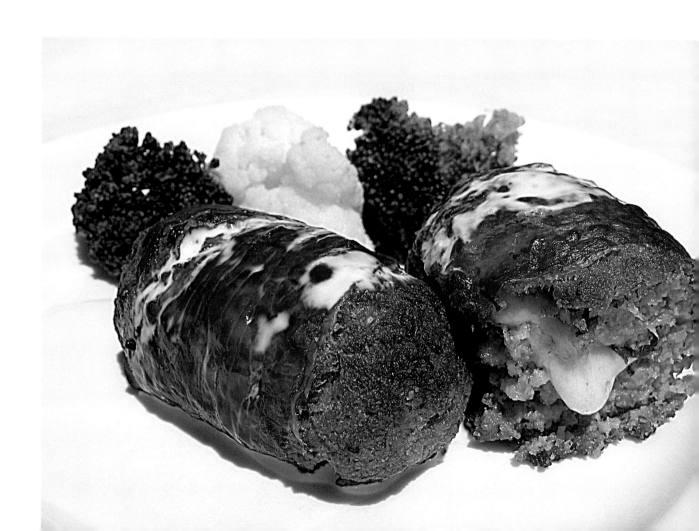

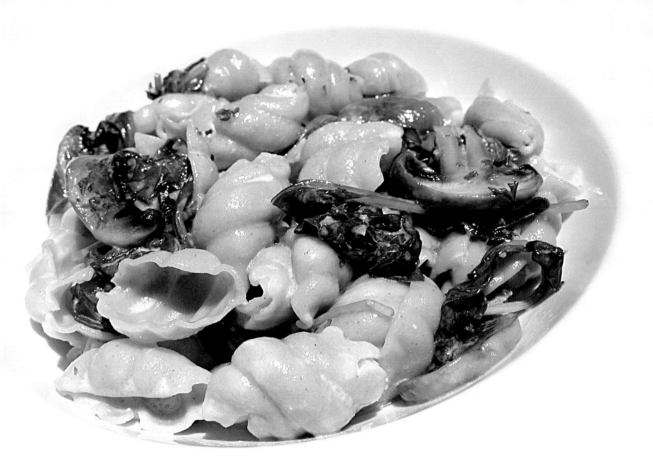

CREAMY MUSHROOM AND BLUE CHEESE PASTA

500g gluten free pasta
2 Tbsp olive oil
2 cloves garlic, crushed
350g mushrooms, sliced
1/2 cup (125ml) reduced fat cream
1/3 cup (85ml) white wine
100g blue vein cheese
3 cups (100g) baby spinach leaves
1/4 cup fresh parsley, chopped
salt, freshly ground black pepper to taste

Cook gluten free pasta in a large pot of boiling water until just tender. Drain, keep warm.

While pasta is cooking, heat olive oil in a heavy-based pan over medium heat. Add crushed garlic and mushrooms, stir until mushrooms are soft. Add cream and wine, simmer, stirring occasionally for 5 to 7 minutes or until liquid has reduced and thickened. Add crumbled blue vein cheese, stir until melted. Remove from heat, stir through cooked pasta, baby spinach leaves, parsley, salt and pepper.

Serves 4

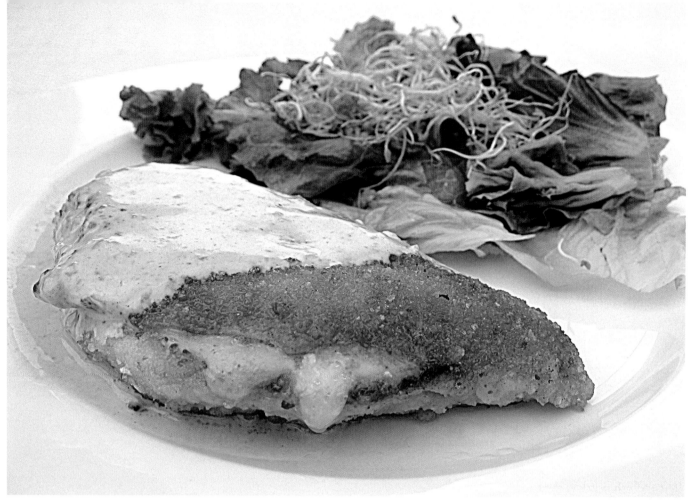

SWISS CHICKEN WITH MUSTARD SAUCE

4 x 150g chicken breasts, skin removed
2 slices (60g) Swiss cheese, cut in half
2 slices (80g) Virginian ham, cut in half
1/4 cup (35g) gluten free cornflour
2 eggs, lightly beaten
1 cup (120g) gluten free breadcrumbs
3 Tbsp canola oil

Mustard sauce
1/2 cup (125ml) reduced fat cream
3 tsp gluten free smooth mild prepared mustard (more if desired)

Cut each chicken breast in half lengthways. Place one slice of cheese, and half slice of ham into the middle of each chicken breast. Set out three shallow bowls. Pour cornflour into one, beaten eggs into another, and pour breadcrumbs into the final bowl. Dip stuffed chicken breasts in cornflour, then in egg, then toss in breadcrumbs. Ensure the chicken has not opened up, keep filling well enclosed within the chicken breast. Repeat for each chicken breast. Heat oil in a non-stick pan over medium-low heat. Cook crumbed chicken fillets until golden brown on both sides and cooked through. Serve topped with mustard sauce.

Mustard sauce: In a small saucepan, combine cream and mustard. Stir over medium heat for 3 to 5 minutes or until sauce has thickened slightly.

Serves 4

VEGETABLE PASTA BAKE

1¹/2 cups (130g) gluten free pasta spirals
2¹/2 cups (400g) pumpkin, cut into 1cm cubes
410g can tomatoes. crushed
1 x 425g can chickpeas
2 medium (300g) zucchini, grated
5 eggs, lightly beaten
¹/2 cup (60g), parmesan cheese, grated
¹/4 cup fresh parsley, chopped
3 tsp ground cumin
1 tsp mustard powder
salt, freshly ground black pepper to taste
¹/2 cup (60g) parmesan cheese, grated, extra
¹/2 cup (60g) gluten free breadcrumbs

Set oven to 180°C. Cook gluten free pasta according to packet directions, until just tender. Set aside. Cook pumpkin pieces in saucepan until just tender.

In a large mixing bowl, combine cooked pasta, pumpkin, tomatoes, chickpeas, zucchini, eggs, parmesan cheese, herbs and spices. Spread into a greased baking dish (21cm x 21cm). Sprinkle evenly with combined extra parmesan cheese and breadcrumbs. Bake in pre-heated oven for 30 minutes or until golden brown.

Serves 6-8

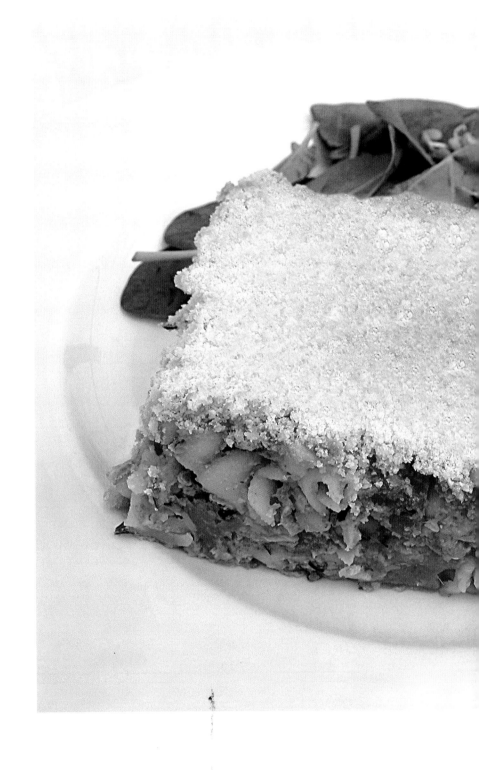

BEEF ROLLS WITH HORSERADISH CRÈME

4 x 150g porterhouse steaks
8 medium (160g) mushrooms, finely chopped
2 cups (70g) fresh baby spinach leaves, finely chopped
2 Tbsp black pitted olives, finely chopped
4 Tbsp cream cheese
salt, freshly ground black pepper to taste

Horseradish crème
1 Tbsp horseradish, grated
squeeze lemon juice
1/4 cup (65ml) reduced fat cream
2 Tbsp fresh parsley, chopped
salt, freshly ground black pepper to taste

Pre-heat oven to 180°C. Grease 26cm x 16cm baking dish. Trim excess fat from meat. Place each steak between two sheets of greaseproof paper, and flatten with a meat tenderiser or rolling pin until steak is approximately 1/3 thickness. Cut each steak in half width-ways (this will make eight square-shaped thin steaks). Set aside.

Mix mushrooms, spinach, olives and cream cheese together in a bowl with a metal spoon until well combined. Add salt and pepper to taste. Place approximately 1 tablespoon of cream cheese mix across the centre of each flattened steak portion. Roll up steak, encasing filling, secure with toothpick. Place in greased baking dish and bake in pre-heated oven for 10 minutes, then cover with foil and bake for further 5 minutes or until cooked through. Remove from heat, serve two rolls per person, topped with prepared horseradish crème.

Horseradish crème: Combine horseradish, cream, lemon juice, parsley, salt and pepper in a small saucepan. Heat gently over medium-low heat, simmering, for 3 to 5 minutes, until thickened slightly. Do not boil.

Serves 4

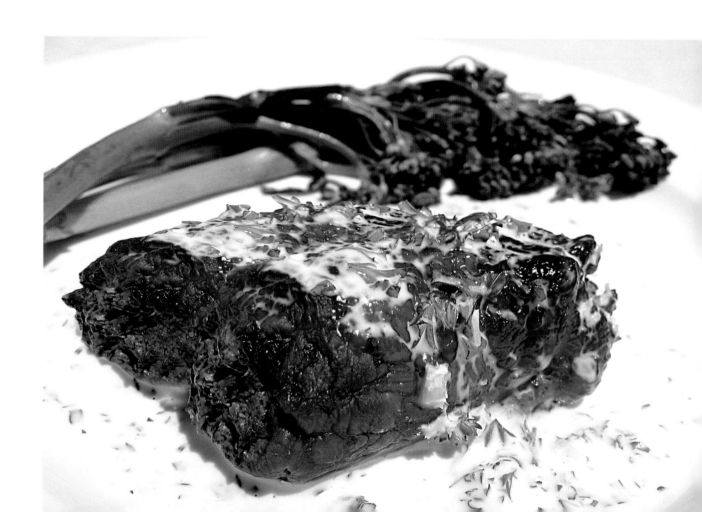

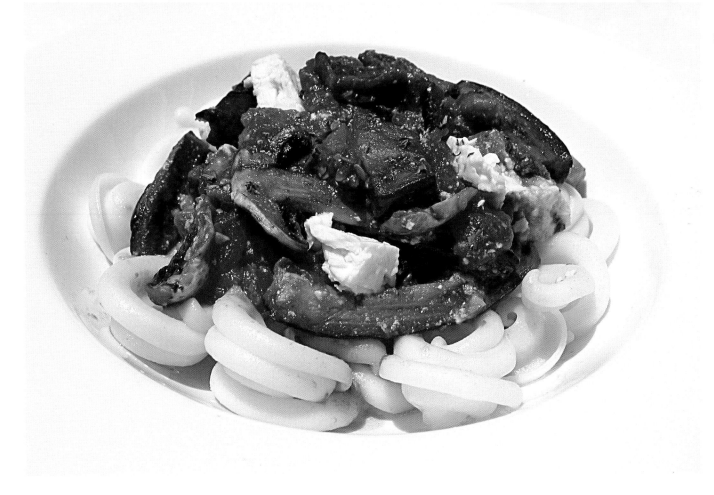

GRILLED EGGPLANT WITH FETTA PASTA

1 large (500g) eggplant
olive oil
500g packet gluten free pasta
150g mushrooms, sliced
2 cloves garlic, crushed
1 Tbsp olive oil
200g fetta cheese
1 cup (275g) canned tomatoes, crushed
1/4 cup continental parsley, finely chopped

Turn grill on to high. Slice eggplant lengthways into 1cm-thick slices. Arrange over baking tray, and brush with olive oil. Heat under the grill until golden brown, then turn to brown other side. Remove from grill, cover with foil to allow eggplant to sweat, set aside for 10 minutes.

Cook gluten free pasta in a large pot of boiling water until just tender. While pasta is cooking, remove foil from eggplant. Cut eggplant into thin strips, 2cm long. In a large heavy-based pan, sauté mushrooms and garlic in olive oil until mushrooms softened and lightly browned. Add fetta cheese, crushed tomatoes, eggplant strips and parsley, stirring to ensure well combined. Finally, add cooked, drained pasta. Stir through gently then serve.

Serves 4

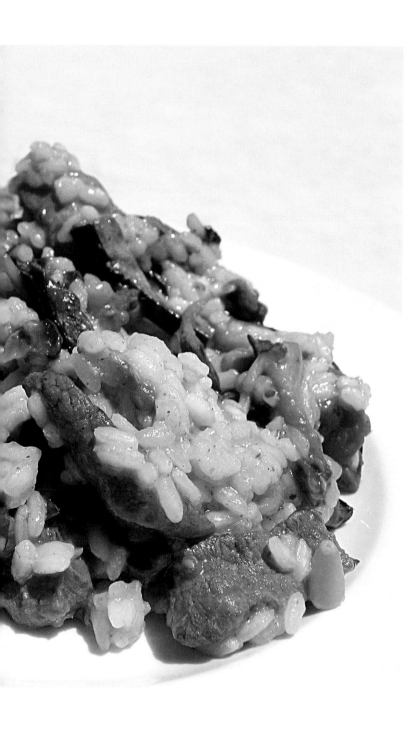

MIDDLE EASTERN PUMPKIN AND LAMB RISOTTO

300g pumpkin, cut into 2cm cubes
olive oil
1 medium (330g) eggplant, cut into 1cm slices
1/3 cup (55g) pine nuts, toasted
1 Tbsp gluten free Middle Eastern spices
3 cloves garlic, crushed
500g lamb strips
9 cups (2250ml) gluten free beef stock
2 1/4 cups (500g) Arborio rice
1/2 cup (60g) parmesan cheese, grated
2 cups (70g) baby spinach leaves

Pre-heat oven to 180°C. Brush diced pumpkin with olive oil, bake in oven for 30 minutes or until tender. Set aside. Brush eggplant slices with olive oil, place in single layer over baking tray. Bake in oven for 30 minutes. Cut into 2cm strips. Set aside. Sprinkle pine nuts over baking tray, heat in oven for 5 minutes, or until golden brown. Set aside. In a medium frying pan, heat garlic and Middle Eastern spice in 1 tablespoon of oil. Add lamb strips and toss through spices, heating until just cooked. Set aside.

Heat beef stock in medium-sized saucepan, keep simmering, covered, over low heat. Combine 1 cup of heated beef stock and rice in a large stockpot. Stir until nearly all of the stock is absorbed. Add another 1/2 cup of heated stock. Continue stirring through rice until all stock absorbed. Repeat this process until all but last 1/2 cup of stock used. Add pumpkin, eggplant, pine nuts, lamb, cheese and spinach leaves. Stir through until well combined. Add remaining stock. Stir until absorbed and rice is tender.

Serves 4-6

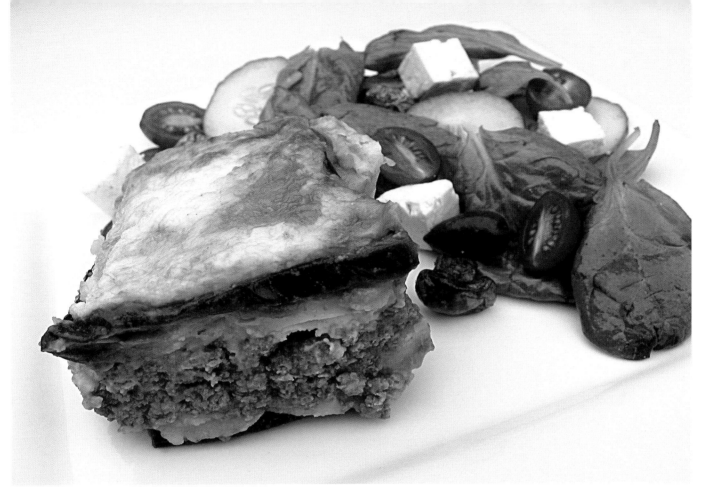

MOUSSAKA

6 medium (1100g) potatoes, peeled
2 large (1000g) eggplant, sliced thinly
2 Tbsp olive oil
2 cloves garlic, crushed
500g lean lamb mince
3/4 cup (190ml) tomato purée
salt, freshly ground black pepper to taste
1 1/2 cups (375ml) reduced fat milk •
3 Tbsp gluten free cornflour
1/2 cup (60g) parmesan cheese, grated

Pre-heat oven to 180°C. Grease a 18cm x 27cm baking dish. In a large saucepan, boil potatoes until just tender. Remove from heat immediately; sit in bowl of cold water to cool. When potatoes have cooled, cut into thin slices. Set aside. Place eggplant in single layers on greased baking trays. Brush with a little olive oil and bake in oven for 10 to 15 minutes or until tender. Remove from oven, set aside.

In a large non-stick pan over medium heat, sauté garlic and lamb mince until browned. Add tomato purée, salt and pepper as desired. Turn down heat to low, simmer for 5 to 10 minutes or until sauce thickens slightly.

In a small mixing bowl, combine 1/4 cup milk with cornflour to form a paste. Add remaining milk, mixing well to ensure evenly combined. Pour into a saucepan, stirring constantly over medium heat until thickened. Do not boil. Add cheese, stir until melted.

Place half of the cooked eggplant slices over the base of baking dish in a single layer. Top with half of the cooked potato slices to make the next layer. Top the potato with all of the cooked lamb sauce. Spread half of the cheese sauce over the lamb. Top with a layer of remaining potato, then eggplant and finally the remaining cheese sauce. Bake in oven for 25 to 30 minutes or until golden brown on top.

Serves 6-8   • See recipe hints p.132

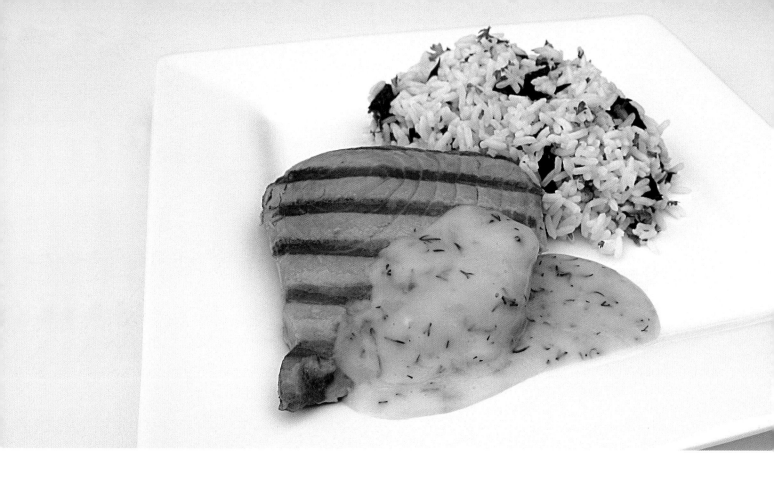

CHARGRILLED FISH STEAKS WITH LEMON DILL SAUCE AND SPINACH RICE

2 egg yolks
1 tsp lemon rind, grated
1 Tbsp lemon juice
60g butter, cubed at room temperature
1¹/2 Tbsp fresh dill, chopped
4 x 200g tuna, marlin or swordfish steaks
1 Tbsp extra virgin olive oil
salt, freshly ground black pepper to taste

Place egg yolks, lemon rind and juice in a small bowl, set over a small saucepan of boiling water. Stir until well combined for 2 minutes. Add small pieces of butter gradually, stirring until sauce thickens. Finally, stir through dill, then set aside, keeping warm.

Heat a chargrill or large heavy-based frying pan on high heat. Brush both sides of fish steak with oil and season lightly with salt and pepper. Add steaks to the chargrill, and reduce heat to medium-high. Cook the steaks for 3 minutes each side, or until cooked to your liking. Serve the cooked fish steaks with prepared warm lemon dill sauce, and spinach rice on the side.

Spinach Rice
6 cups (200g) baby spinach leaves
2 cloves garlic, crushed
1/2 cup (125ml) olive oil
1/4 cup (60ml) lemon juice
4 cups (800g) cooked long grain white rice
1/4 cup fresh parsley, chopped
1 Tbsp lemon rind, finely grated
salt, freshly ground black pepper to taste

In a large frying pan, sauté baby spinach leaves in garlic, olive oil and lemon juice until spinach just wilted. Add cooked rice, parsley, and lemon rind. Taste, season with salt and pepper. Stir until well combined and heated through.

Serves 4

ROASTED FIELD MUSHROOMS STUFFED WITH TANDOORI RISOTTO

4 cups (1000ml) hot gluten free vegetable stock
1 1/3 cups (300g) Arborio rice
1/3 cup (85ml) tomato purée
1 Tbsp fresh coriander, finely chopped
1 tsp sweet paprika
1/2 tsp chilli powder
1 tsp garam masala
1/2 cup (125g) gluten free natural yoghurt
salt, freshly ground black pepper to taste
6 large (750g) field mushrooms
gluten free natural yoghurt, extra

Pre-heat oven to 180°C. Heat vegetable stock in a large saucepan. Add rice, tomato purée, herbs and spices. Cook covered, stirring regularly, over medium heat until all liquid is absorbed, and rice is tender. Let stand for 5 minutes. Stir through yoghurt, salt and pepper to taste.

Use a damp cloth to wipe clean outer surface of mushroom. Remove stem. Set out on flat baking tray. Place spoonfuls of tandoori risotto mixture evenly over four mushrooms. Bake in pre-heated oven for 15 to 20 minutes or until mushrooms softened. Remove from oven, top with a spoonful of extra natural yoghurt.

Serves 6

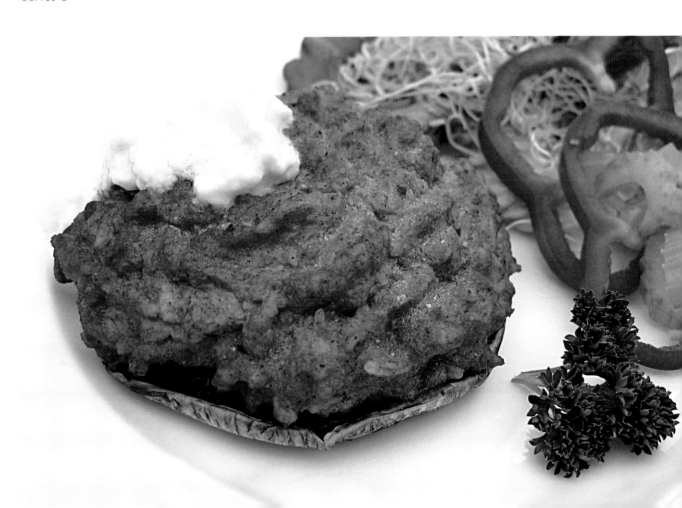

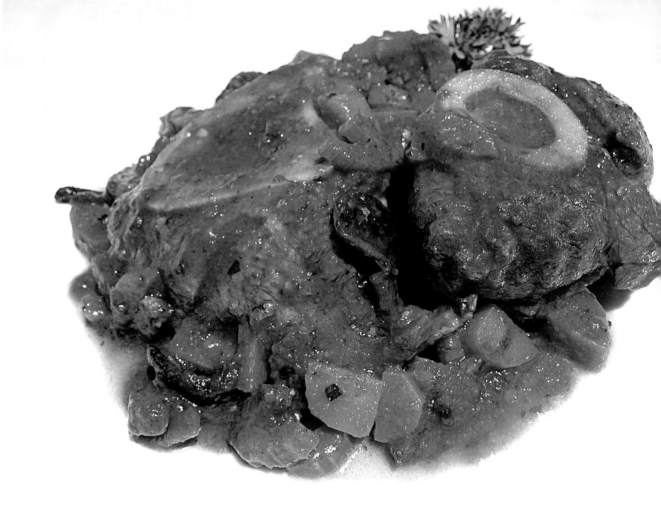

OSSO BUCCO

4 Tbsp gluten free cornflour
salt, freshly ground black pepper
8 x 150g osso bucco pieces
4 Tbsp olive oil
3 small (360g) carrots, diced
6 medium (120g) mushrooms, sliced
2 (180g) sticks celery, sliced
2 whole small onions, peeled
2 cloves garlic, crushed
1 tsp chilli flakes (or to taste)
3 cups (750ml) gluten free beef stock
1 1/2 cups (375ml) tomato purée
1/4 cup fresh parsley, chopped
1 Tbsp dried Italian herbs
1 Tbsp fresh oregano

In a shallow bowl, combine cornflour, salt and pepper. Toss each piece of meat in flour. In a large non-stick stockpot, heat 2 tablespoons of olive oil. Sauté half the floured osso bucco pieces for 2 to 3 minutes, turn, browning both sides. Remove from pan, repeat for the second batch with remaining olive oil. Remove meat pieces from pan, set aside. Add carrot, mushrooms, celery, whole onions, garlic and chilli to pot, tossing through the meat juices in the pan. Add the meat back to the pot with vegetables. Cover with beef stock, tomato purée and herbs. Stir until well combined. Reduce heat, simmer uncovered for 40 to 50 minutes, stirring occasionally. Sauce will reduce and thicken. Discard whole onions prior to serving.

Serves 4

MEXICAN BEEF GORDITAS

8 maize tortillas
1 can (400g) red kidney beans
3/4 cup canned tomatoes, crushed
1 clove garlic, crushed
1 1/2 tsp sweet paprika
1 1/2 tsp ground cumin
1 tsp cayenne pepper
500g lean beef steak, cut into strips
2 tsp canola oil
1 medium (150g) zucchini, cut into strips
1/2 red (150g) capsicum, sliced into 2cm strips
1/2 iceberg lettuce, washed, shredded
1/3 cup (50g) peanuts, crushed
1 1/4 cups (125g) tasty cheese, grated

Pre-heat oven to 180°C. Wrap tortillas in foil and heat for 20 minutes (or place maize tortillas on a clean tea towel. Sprinkle a little water over the tortillas, and heat in microwave for 1 minute and 20 seconds on high just prior to serving).
Place kidney beans, crushed tomatoes, garlic and spices in a food processor. Process for 2 minutes, or until evenly puréed. In a medium frying pan over medium-low heat, sauté beef steak in canola oil until just browned. Pour kidney bean sauce over steak strips. Add zucchini and capsicum and simmer over low heat for 5 to 7 minutes.

Place a little shredded lettuce on warmed tortillas. Top with beef mixture, sprinkle with 1 to 2 teaspoons of crushed peanuts and 2 tablespoons of grated cheese. Fold to encase filling and serve immediately.

Serves 4

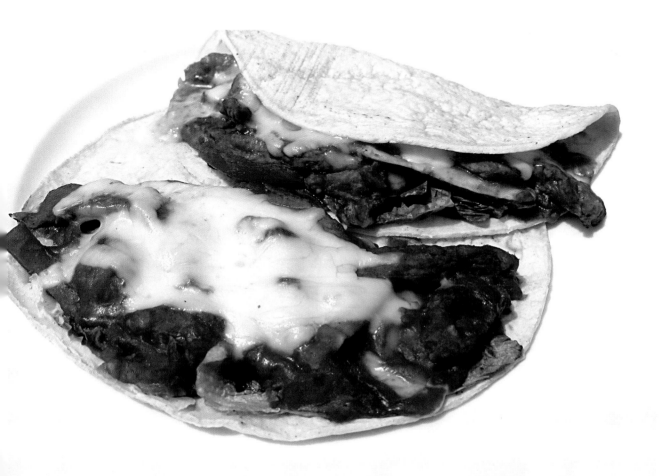

CHICKEN AND VEGETABLE CURRY

4 cloves garlic, crushed
1 Tbsp garam masala
1 Tbsp ground cumin
2 tsp ground turmeric
1/2 tsp chilli powder (adjust according to taste)
1/4 cup (55g) brown sugar
1 Tbsp sesame oil
4 x 200g chicken thigh fillets
3 medium (240g) Roma tomatoes, chopped
1 medium (150g) zucchini, halved and sliced
250g cauliflower, cut into 2cm florettes
250g pumpkin, cut into 2cm pieces
1/2 cup (125ml) water

In a large stockpot, sauté garlic, spices and sugar in sesame oil over medium heat to develop flavour. Add chicken fillets, tomatoes, zucchini, cauliflower, pumpkin and water. Turn heat down to medium low, cover, stirring occasionally until chicken and vegetables tender, and sauce thickened. Serve with cooked rice.

Serves 4

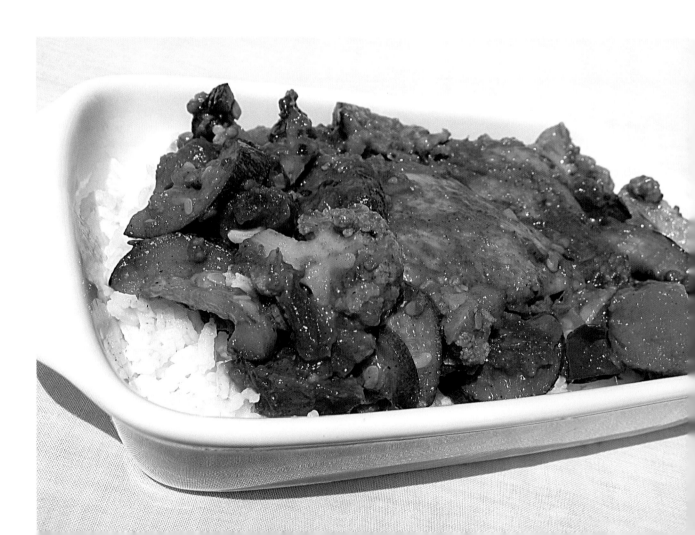

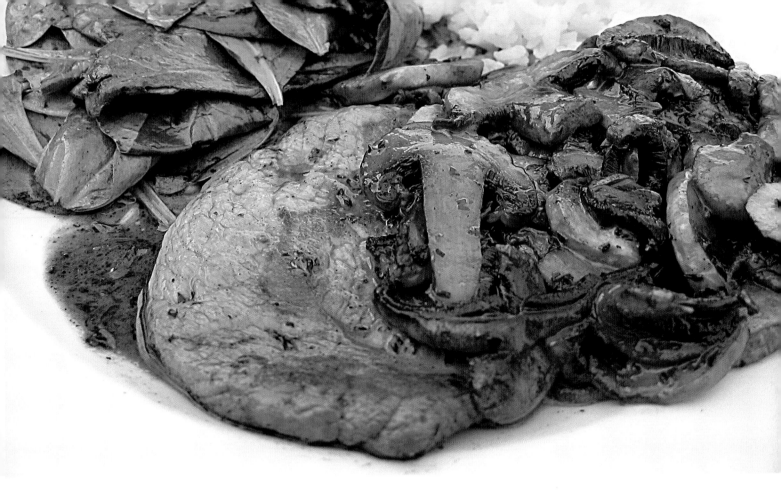

VEAL STEAKS WITH MUSHROOM SAUCE

1 1/2 Tbsp (30g) butter
500g mushrooms, sliced
1/2 cup (125ml) strong gluten free beef stock
3 Tbsp fresh parsley, chopped
1/2 cup (125ml) reduced fat cream
salt, freshly ground black pepper to taste
2 Tbsp olive oil
4 x 180g veal steaks

In a small frying pan, melt butter and add sliced mushrooms. Cook gently over medium-low heat until mushrooms are soft. Add beef stock, parsley, cream, salt and pepper. Cook uncovered, simmering, until sauce thickens slightly. Reduce heat, keep warm.

In a large frying pan, heat olive oil. Add veal steaks to hot pan, cook 3 to 5 minutes, then turn. Cook for a further 3 to 5 minutes (or to personal preference). Serve topped with prepared mushroom sauce.

Serves 4

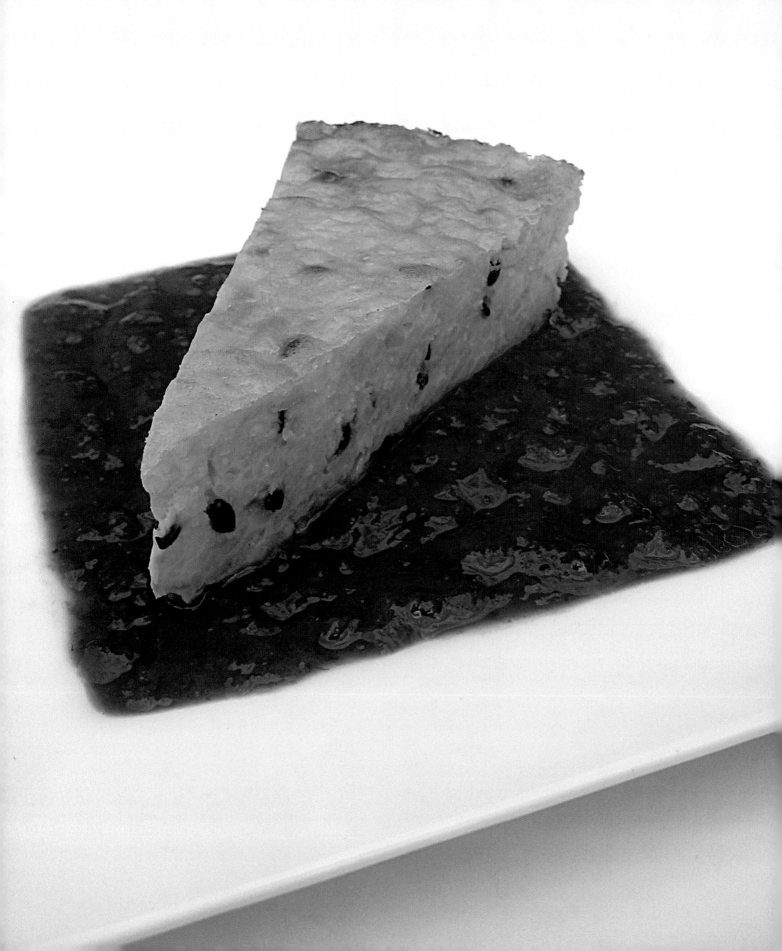

desserts

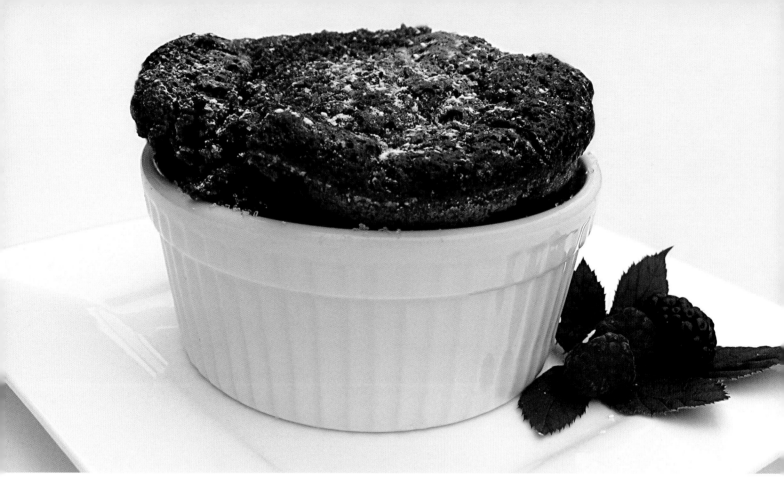

CHOCOLATE SOUFFLÉ

butter for greasing
6 Tbsp sugar
220g good quality dark chocolate, broken into pieces
1/2 cup (125ml) reduced fat thickened cream
6 eggs, separated
2/3 cup (100g) gluten free cornflour
3/4 cup (165g) caster sugar
1/4 cup (55g) brown sugar, firmly packed
1/2 cup (125ml) reduced fat milk •
pure icing sugar, sifted

Pre-heat oven to 180°C. Grease six 1-cup capacity soufflé dishes. Place 1 tablespoon sugar in each dish, shake around to coat greased butter coating. Discard excess.

Place chocolate and cream in a heatproof bowl set over a saucepan of simmering water. Heat, stirring constantly, until mixture is smooth. Remove bowl from pan and set aside. Place egg yolks and caster sugar in a clean bowl, and beat with electric beaters until pale, thick and creamy. Gradually, beat in cornflour, caster sugar, brown sugar and milk until well combined. Pour egg yolk mixture into a medium-sized saucepan. Cook over a medium heat, stirring constantly, for 5 minutes or until mixture thickens. Remove from heat and stir in chocolate mixture.

Place egg whites in a bowl and beat with clean electric beaters until stiff peaks form. Fold egg whites into chocolate mixture. Fill soufflé dishes to approximately 1cm below the top rim of soufflé dish. Place dishes on a baking tray and bake in pre-heated oven for 20 to 25 minutes or until soufflés have risen well. Dust with icing sugar, and serve immediately, as they will sink on standing.

Alternative flavours:
Mocha: add 1 Tbsp instant coffee powder to melted chocolate and cream mix
Passionfruit: replace chocolate with 1/2 cup passionfruit pulp
Choc Mint: replace dark chocolate with gluten free peppermint-filled chocolate

Serves 6 • See recipe hints p.132

INDIVIDUAL IRISH CREAM DELIGHTS

3/4 cup (185ml) reduced fat milk •
1 1/4 cup (310ml) reduced fat cream
1/2 cup (75g) brown sugar
1/2 cup (125ml) Irish cream liqueur
3 Tbsp gluten free cornflour
1/4 cup (65ml) reduced fat milk, extra •

Heat milk, cream and brown sugar in saucepan over medium heat until almost boiling. Stir in Irish cream liqueur. Mix cornflour in extra milk to form smooth paste. Add slowly into warm Irish cream mix, stirring constantly to ensure smooth consistency. Heat, stirring constantly for 5 minutes or until thickened. Do not boil. Pour into four individual dessert dishes. Allow to cool slightly, then refrigerate for 3 to 4 hours or until set. Decorate prior to serving.

Hint: If lactose intolerant, this dessert may be unsuitable. Half-serves may be tolerated with • recipe modifications.

Serves 4   • See recipe hints p.132

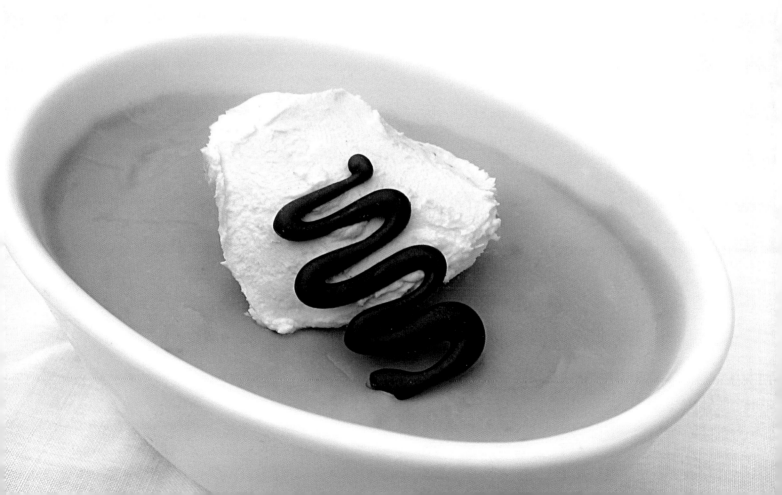

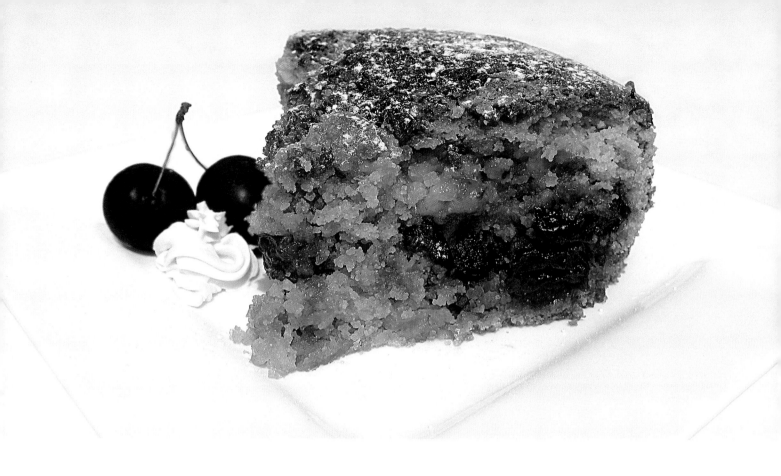

BAKED CHERRY PUDDING

125g butter
1 cup (170g) rice flour
1/2 cup (75g) gluten free cornflour
1/2 cup (90g) potato flour •
1 tsp bicarb soda
2 tsp gluten free baking powder
1 tsp xanthan gum (optional)•
1 cup (220g) sugar
3/4 cup (165ml) reduced fat milk •
1 egg
1 tsp vanilla essence
410g canned pitted cherries•, drained, 1/2 cup liquid reserved
1/4 cup (55g) sugar, extra

Pre-heat oven to 160°C. Grease a 15cm x 15cm baking dish. Melt butter and pour into base of baking dish. Sift flours, bicarb soda, baking powder and xanthan gum three times. Add sugar, milk, egg and vanilla essence into sifted flours. Use electric beaters to mix well. Pour over melted butter – do not mix. Pour the cherries and reserved liquid over the flour mixture – do not mix. Sprinkle extra sugar over the dessert and bake for 50 minutes or until cooked. If making individual puddings, bake for 20 to 25 minutes. Let stand for 5 minutes before serving.

Serves 6   • • • See recipe hints p.132

LAYERED TAHITIAN LIME CHEESECAKE

1 pkt (200g) plain gluten free sweet biscuits
60g butter, melted
1/2 cup (125ml) boiling water
1 1/2 Tbsp gelatine
500g reduced fat cream cheese
1 x 400g can sweetened condensed skim milk
1/3 cup (85ml) coconut liqueur (e.g. Malibu)
2 1/2 Tbsp lime juice
rind of one lime, finely grated
1 to 2 drops green food colouring

Crush biscuits to form fine crumbs. Add melted butter, stir until well combined. Press evenly into the base of a 19cm springform tin. Combine boiling water and gelatine in a small heat-proof bowl. Set bowl over larger bowl of boiling water, stirring constantly until all the gelatine has dissolved. In food processor, combine cream cheese, sweetened condensed milk, and gelatine. Process for 1 minute. Pour out half of the filling mixture into a separate bowl (should be approximately 500ml). Stir into this bowl coconut liqueur. Mix well with a spoon until evenly combined. Pour over prepared base, and place in freezer for 10 minutes.

Add lime rind, juice and green food colouring to filling mix remaining in food processing bowl. Blend on high setting for further 30 seconds until well combined. Remove cheesecake from freezer, should be just set. Pour lime filling over coconut layer. Place in refrigerator and allow to set for 2 to 3 hours.

Hint: If lactose intolerant, this dessert is unsuitable. Half-serves may be tolerated.

Serves 10-12

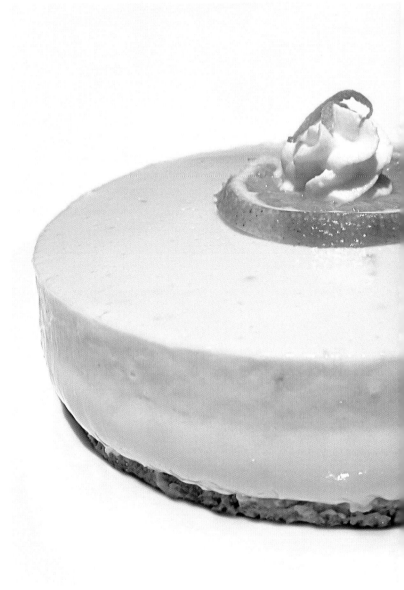

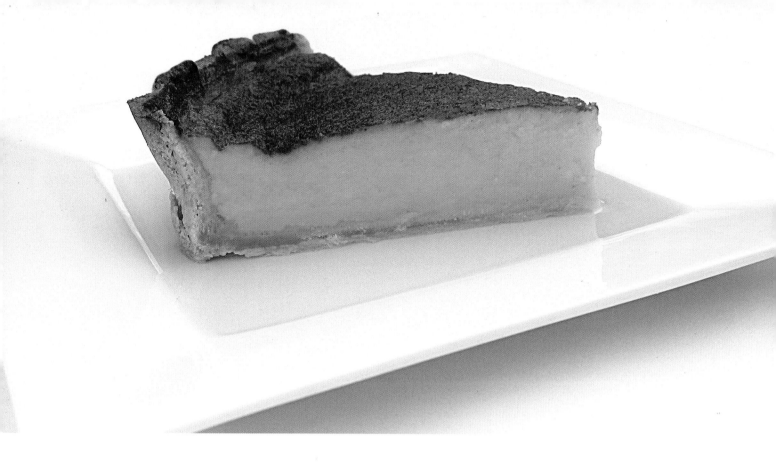

LEMON TART

Pastry
1 cup (130g) fine rice flour •
1/2 cup (75g) gluten free cornflour
1/2 cup (45g) soy flour •
1 tsp xanthan gum (optional) •
1/4 cup (55g) caster sugar
160g butter
6 Tbsp (120ml) iced water

Filling
3/4 cup (165g) caster sugar
200g mascarpone cheese
1 Tbsp lemon rind, finely grated
2/3 cup (165ml) fresh lemon juice
4 eggs
pure icing sugar, to dust

Pastry: Pre-heat oven to 180°C Grease 23cm fluted tart dish. Sift flours and xanthan gum three times into a bowl. Combine sifted flours, sugar and butter in food processor. Process until it resembles fine breadcrumbs. While the motor is running, add iced water (tablespoon at a time) to allow mixture to form soft dough. Knead on gluten-free cornfloured bench. Wrap in plastic wrap and refrigerate for 30 minutes before rolling to use. Roll pastry 2mm thick between two sheets of non-stick bake wrap large enough to line 23cm flan tin. Place in prepared flan tin, trim edges to neaten. Blind bake (see hint) in pre-heated oven for 10 minutes or until lightly browned.

Filling: Turn oven temperature down to 160°C. Using electric beaters, combine sugar, mascarpone cheese, lemon rind and juice in a small bowl. Add eggs, one at a time, beating well between additions. Pour into pre-cooked base. Bake in reduced temperature oven for 30 to 35 minutes or until set. Allow to cool in dish before serving.

Hint: To blind bake, place pastry in the pan, cover with a sheet of greaseproof paper then fill with uncooked rice grains. The rice acts as a weight to prevent the case from rising up during baking.

Serves 8-10   • See recipe hints p.132

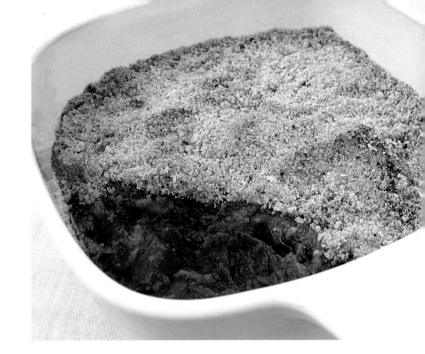

MIXED BERRY WHIP

1 can (375ml) reduced fat evaporated milk
4 egg whites, at room temperature
2/3 cup (150g) caster sugar
2 tsp vanilla essence
1 x 410g can mixed berries in syrup, drained

Place the can of evaporated milk in freezer until just about to freeze. (You will feel ice crystals in the can when you shake it.) In a medium mixing bowl, use electric beaters to beat egg whites until soft peaks form. Gradually add sugar, continue beating until stiff peaks form. Beat chilled evaporated milk and vanilla essence with electric beaters until mixture thick and foamy, and doubled in volume. Fold beaten egg whites and berries into whipped evaporated milk. Pour into container suitable for freezing, freeze for 2 to 3 hours or until firm. Serve on the same day whip is prepared as it may separate over time.

Hint: If lactose intolerant, this dessert is unsuitable. Ingredients cannot be substituted.

Serves 4-6

RHUBARB AND RASPBERRY CRUMBLE

1 bunch (500g) rhubarb sticks, cut into 3cm pieces
1/2 cup (110g) sugar
1 x 410g can raspberries in syrup, drained
1/4 cup (40g) pure icing sugar
3/4 cup (130g) rice flour
1/2 cup (75g) brown sugar
2 Tbsp desiccated coconut
60g butter, at room temperature, cubed

Pre-heat oven to 180°C. Grease a 20cm square baking dish. In a medium saucepan, add rhubarb pieces and sugar. Cook in water until just tender, then drain. Add cooked rhubarb, raspberries and icing sugar to a medium bowl. Stir until well combined, then spoon into the base of greased baking dish.

In a small bowl, combine rice flour, sugar and coconut. Rub in butter until mixture resembles fine breadcrumbs. Sprinkle evenly over rhubarb/raspberry mix. Bake in pre-heated oven for 30 minutes or until golden brown.

Serves 8

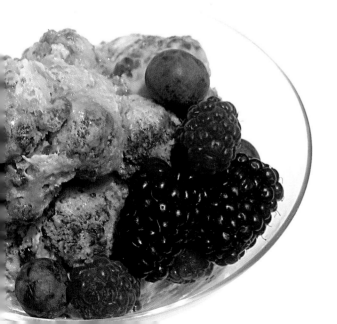

STEAMED BANANA PUDDING WITH CARAMEL SAUCE

100g butter, room temperature
3/4 cup (165g) caster sugar
1 tsp vanilla essence
2 eggs
2 (260g) bananas, mashed
1/3 cup (50g) gluten free cornflour
3/4 cup (130g) rice flour
1/2 cup (50g) soy flour •
1 tsp bicarb soda
2 tsp gluten free baking powder
1 tsp xanthan gum (optional) •

Caramel sauce
1/2 cup (125ml) reduced fat cream
1/2 cup (110g) brown sugar, firmly packed

Grease a 15cm pudding basin. Line base with greaseproof paper.

Use electric beaters to beat butter, sugar and vanilla in a medium bowl until well combined. Add eggs, one at a time, beating well between each addition. Add mashed banana, mix well. Into a medium bowl, sift flours, bicarb soda, baking powder and xanthan gum three times. Add sifted flours to creamed banana mixture, stir well with a wooden spoon to gently combine. Spoon into greased pudding basin, smooth the surface. Place pudding basin into a large stockpot. Fill stockpot with boiling water so that it covers halfway up the basin. Cook over medium-low heat for 1 to 11/4 hours, or until pudding cooked. Check if cooked by inserting a skewer, it should come out clean. Top with caramel sauce.

Caramel sauce: Combine cream and sugar in a small saucepan. Stir constantly over medium-low heat until sugar combined and sauce thickens slightly.

Serves 6   • See recipe hints p.132

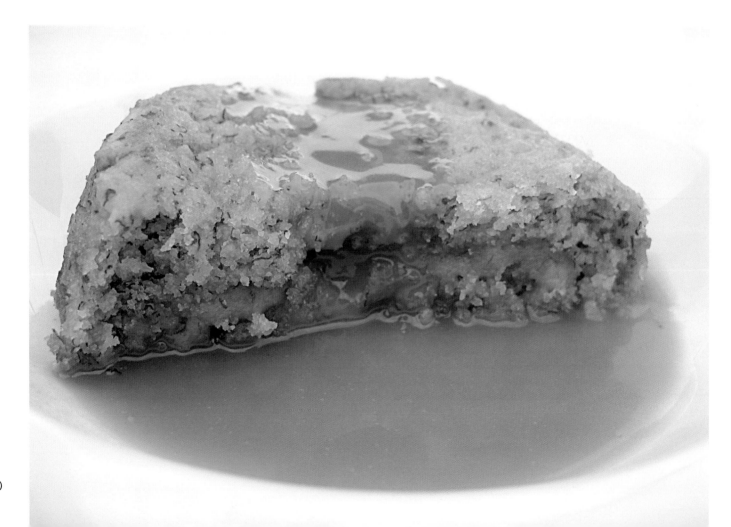

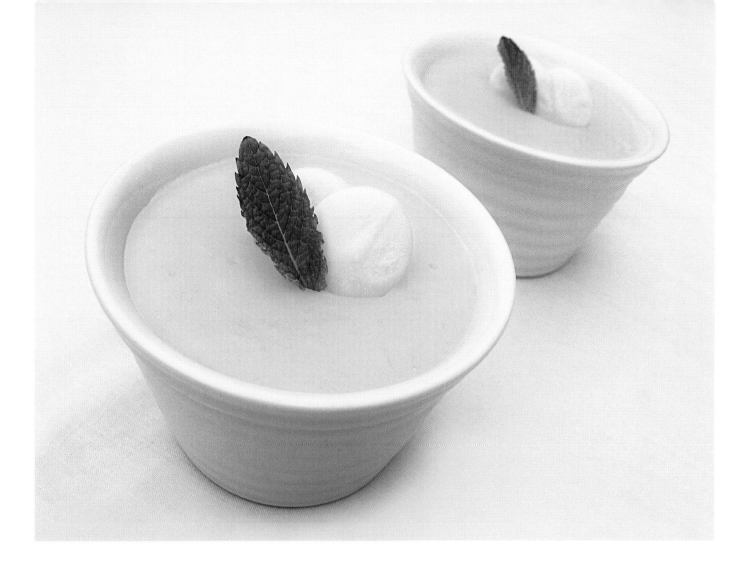

WHITE CHOC MINT POTS

3/4 cup (185ml) reduced fat milk •
1 1/4 cups (310ml) reduced fat cream
1/2 cup (110g) caster sugar
1/4 tsp (15 drops) peppermint essence (more to taste)
3-4 drops green food colouring
100g white chocolate buttons
3 Tbsp gluten free cornflour
1/4 cup (65ml) reduced fat milk, extra •

Heat milk, cream, sugar, peppermint essence and green colouring in saucepan over medium heat until almost boiling. Do not boil. Add chocolate buttons, stir until completely melted. Mix cornflour in extra milk to form smooth paste. Add slowly into chocolate cream mix, stirring constantly to ensure smooth consistency. Heat, stirring, for 5 minutes or until thickened. Pour into four individual dessert dishes. Allow to cool slightly then refrigerate for 3 to 4 hours or until set. Decorate prior to serving.

Hint: If lactose intolerant, this dessert may be unsuitable. Half-serves may be tolerated with • recipe modifications.

Serves 4   • See recipe hints p.132

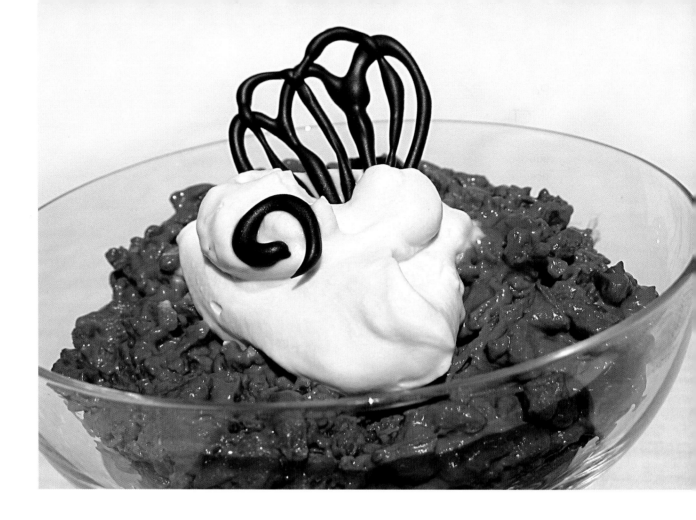

CHOCOLATE RICE WITH SAMBUCA CREAM

3 cups (750ml) reduced fat milk •
200ml reduced fat cream
1/2 cup (110g) medium grain white rice
1/4 cup (55g) caster sugar
120g good quality dark chocolate

Sambuca Cream
1/2 cup (125ml) thickened cream
1 Tbsp Sambuca liqueur

Combine milk, cream, rice, sugar and chocolate in a medium saucepan. Cook over medium-high heat, uncovered, stirring constantly until mixture comes to the boil. Reduce heat to medium-low, stirring regularly and cook until rice is tender, and mixture is thick and creamy. This will take approximately 50 to 60 minutes. Remove from heat, portion out into individual serving dishes and refrigerate. Serve topped with Sambuca cream.

Sambuca cream: Mix cream and Sambuca in small bowl. Dollop on cooled chocolate rice prior to serving.

Hint: If lactose intolerant, this dessert may be unsuitable. Half-serves may be tolerated with • recipe modifications.

Serves 4   • See recipe hints p.132

CINNAMON PANNA COTTA WITH BANANA REDUCTION

1 2/3 cups (400ml) reduced fat cream
1/2 cup (125ml) reduced fat milk •
1/2 cup (110g) caster sugar
1 tsp ground cinnamon
1 tsp vanilla essence
1 Tbsp boiling water
2 1/4 tsp gelatine
2 ripe (260g) bananas
2 tsp brown sugar
cinnamon sticks for decoration

Grease four 1/2 cup (125ml) dariole moulds. Heat cream, milk, sugar, cinnamon and vanilla essence in a medium-sized saucepan over low heat. Cook, stirring regularly for 20 minutes. Do not boil. Remove from heat. Combine boiling water and gelatine in a small heat-proof bowl. Set bowl over larger bowl of boiling water, stirring constantly until all gelatine dissolved. Whisk gelatine into cream mixture. Pour this mixture into a medium bowl. Fill a large bowl with ice cubes. Place the bowl of cream mixture on top of the ice-filled bowl. Whisk every few minutes for approximately 10 minutes. Mixture will thicken as it cools. When it is of a consistency that will coat the back of a wooden spoon, pour into greased moulds. Refrigerate for 2 to 3 hours.

To serve, dip each mould into bowl of hot water for a few seconds, then turn out onto serving plates. Decorate with banana reduction and cinnamon.

Banana Reduction: Fork-mash bananas together with sugar in a bowl until smooth and even in consistency.

Hint: If lactose intolerant, this dessert may be unsuitable. Half-serves may be tolerated with • recipe modifications.

Serves 4   • See recipe hints p.132

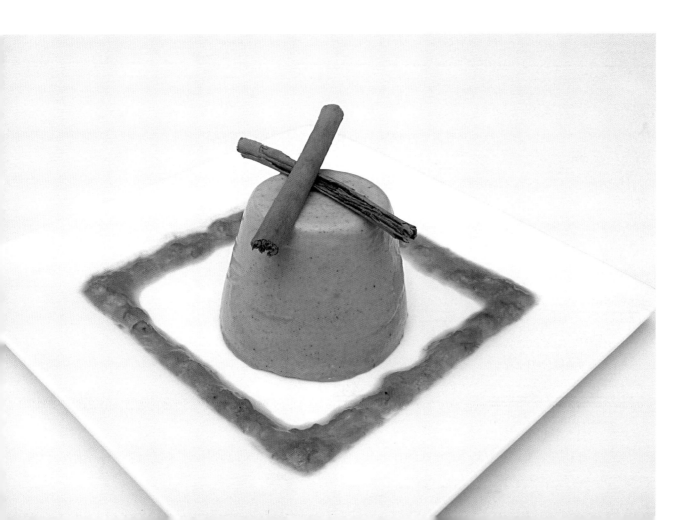

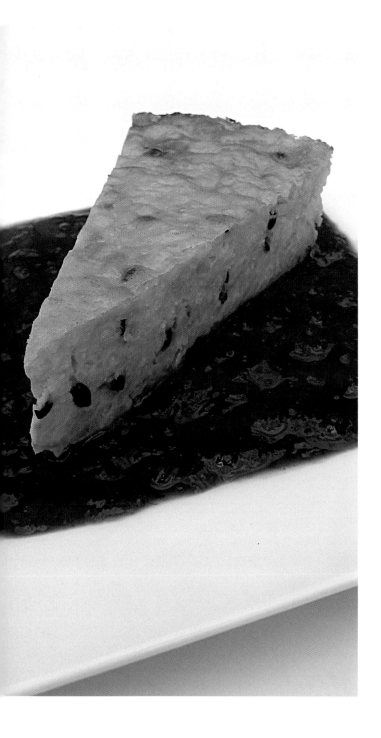

PASSIONFRUIT AND RASPBERRY RICE TART

1 cup (220g) medium grain white rice
1/4 cup (55g) sugar
6 cups boiling water
4 Tbsp (50g) gluten free custard powder
3 eggs, lightly beaten
3/4 cup (190ml) reduced fat cream
3 x 170g cans passionfruit pulp

Raspberry Sauce
2 x (425g) cans raspberries, drained
1/2 cup (125ml) reserved juice
2 Tbsp pure icing sugar
(or 1 cup commercially prepared gluten free raspberry sauce)

Pre-heat oven to 160°C. Grease a 23cm flan dish. Cook rice with sugar in water until tender. Rinse under cold water to cool. Mix custard powder, eggs, cream and passionfruit pulp in a medium mixing bowl. Stir in cooked rice until well combined. Pour into a prepared flan dish. Bake in pre-heated oven for 35 to 40 minutes or until just set. Allow to cool to room temperature, then refrigerate for 2 to 3 hours. Remove from refrigerator 30 minutes prior to serving.

Raspberry sauce: Blend raspberries, juice and icing sugar with hand-held blender until even in consistency. Pour over plate and top with passionfruit rice tart.

Serves 8-10

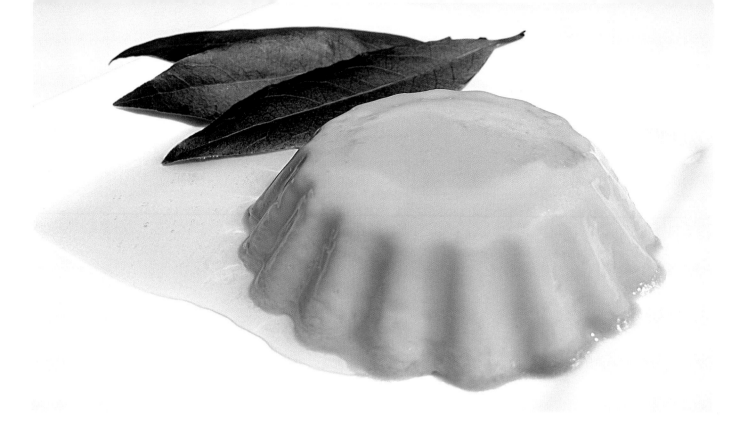

VANILLA BAVAROIS WITH GREEN TEA SYRUP

3 egg yolks, at room temperature
1 cup (220g) caster sugar
1 cup (250ml) reduced fat milk •
1 vanilla bean, split and seeded
2 tsp vanilla essence
2 Tbsp boiling water
1 Tbsp gelatine
1 cup (250ml) thickened cream

Green Tea Syrup
1/2 tsp vanilla essence
2 Tbsp caster sugar
1/2 cup (125ml) green tea (made up from 6 green tea bags)

Grease six 1/2 cup (125ml) dariole moulds. Use electric beaters to beat egg yolks and sugar in a medium mixing bowl. Beat until mixture is thick and pale, approximately 2 to 3 minutes. Set aside.

Heat milk, vanilla bean and essence over low heat in a saucepan. Whisk egg mixture into warm milk. Stir over very low heat continuously with a wooden spoon for 5 minutes. Do not boil. When mixture has thickened, remove from heat.

In a small bowl, combine boiling water and gelatine. Set bowl over a larger bowl of boiling water, stirring constantly until all the gelatine has dissolved. Whisk this into milk. Pour this mixture into a medium bowl. Fill a large bowl with ice cubes. Place the bowl of vanilla mixture on top of the ice-filled bowl. Whisk every few minutes, mixture will thicken as it cools. Allow to cool to a consistency that will coat the back of a wooden spoon.

Beat cream with electric beaters until stiff. Fold vanilla mixure into whipped cream until well combined. Spoon evenly into greased moulds. Cover and refrigerate for 2 to 3 hours. To serve, dip each mould into bowl of hot water for a few seconds, then invert onto plate. Drizzle with green tea syrup prior to serving.

Green Tea Syrup: Combine vanilla essence, sugar and tea in a small saucepan. Stir regularly over medium-low heat until sugar dissolved and syrup thickened, approximately 5 to 6 minutes. Allow to cool to room temperature.

Hint: If lactose intolerant, this dessert may be unsuitable. Half-serves may be tolerated with • recipe modifications.

Serves 6   • See recipe hints p.132

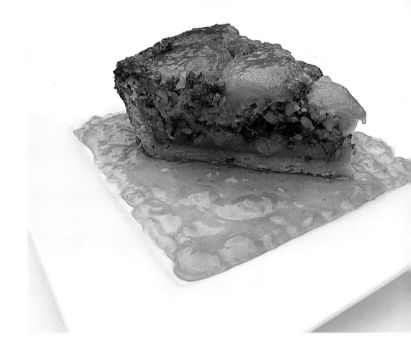

APRICOT AND PISTACHIO RISOTTO

1 1/2 cups (330g) Arborio rice
3/4 cup (165g) caster sugar
4 cups (1000ml) reduced fat milk •
1 cup (250ml) reduced fat cream
2 tsp vanilla essence
1 x 425g canned apricots•, chopped, nectar reserved
1/3 cup (40g) pistachio nuts, crushed

Place rice, sugar, milk, cream, vanilla essence and reserved apricot nectar into a medium saucepan. Bring to the boil, stirring regularly. Reduce heat to simmer, stir regularly (approximately 1 to 1 1/4 hours) until liquid is absorbed and rice is tender. Add extra milk if required. Stir in apricots. Serve with sprinkled pistachio nuts, warm or cooled to room temperature.

Serves 6   • • See recipe hints p.132

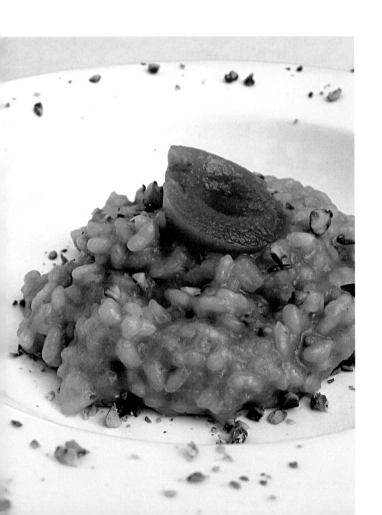

APRICOT AND ALMOND FLAN

Pastry
See recipe page 88 (for lemon tart)

Filling
60g butter
2/3 cup (150g) caster sugar
4 eggs
2 Tbsp gluten free custard powder
2 cups (200g) ground almonds
16 apricot• halves, canned in light syrup, drained
3 Tbsp apricot jam

Pre-heat oven to 180°C.
Pastry: Make as per directions on page 88. Set blind-baked pastry case aside.

Filling: Turn oven down to 160°C. In a large mixing bowl, use electric beaters to cream butter and sugar. Add eggs, one at a time, beating well between additions. Add custard powder and ground almonds. Beat until well combined. Pour mixture over cooked pastry base. Arrange apricot halves on top of filling in circular pattern. Bake in pre-heated oven for 40 to 45 minutes or until golden brown. Brush with warm sieved apricot jam to glaze.

Serves 8-10   • See recipe hints p.132

TROPICAL TANGO BANANA FRITTERS

1 cup (120g) gluten free breadcrumbs
4 Tbsp brown sugar
3 tsp ground cinnamon
2 eggs
1/2 tsp pure icing sugar
4 small bananas, peeled
2 Tbsp (40g) butter
gluten free vanilla ice cream •
1/2 cup (100g) canned pineapple,
    crushed, drained
pulp of 2 passionfruit

Pre-heat oven to 150°C. Combine breadcrumbs,
sugar, and cinnamon on a large plate. Beat
eggs lightly with icing sugar in a shallow
bowl. Halve bananas lengthways, dip in egg
and then toss in breadcrumb mixture, coating
banana well. Heat 1 tablespoon of butter in
a frying pan over medium-low heat. Add half
banana pieces, cook 3 to 4 minutes each
side, until golden brown. Transfer to baking
tray and place in pre-heated oven to keep
warm. Cook remaining banana halves.
Place two cooked halves of banana along the
sides of a serving dish. Fill centre of serving
dish with scoops of ice cream, topped with
2 tablespoons of crushed pineapple and a
drizzle of passionfruit pulp. Serve immediately.

Serves 4   • See recipe hints p.132

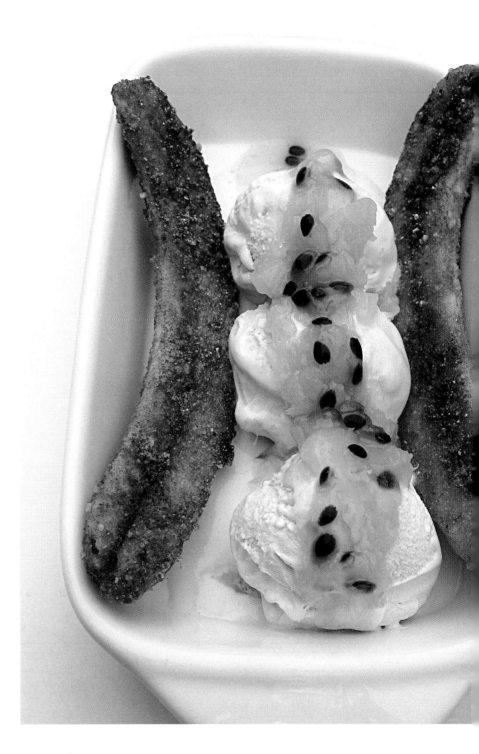

BLUEBERRY PANCAKES

2 eggs
1¹/2 cups (375 ml) milk •
1 cup (170g) rice flour
¹/2 cup (75g) corn flour
¹/2 cup (45g) soy flour •
²/3 cup (150g) firmly packed brown sugar
3 tsp gluten free baking powder
1 tsp xanthan gum (optional) •
3 Tbsp (60g) butter, melted
1 x 150g punnet blueberries

Whisk together egg and milk in a small jug. Sift flours, sugar, baking powder and xanthan gum three times into a large mixing bowl. Make a well in the centre, pour in egg and milk mixture slowly, mixing well. Gradually draw in flour to make a smooth batter. Stir in melted butter, cover and set aside for 15 minutes. Heat a large non-stick frying pan over medium heat, spray with cooking spray. Add enough batter to pan to form 10cm diameter pancake. Cook for 1 minute or until it starts to set. Sprinkle eight blueberries over each and cook for a further 2 minutes. Flip and cook for further 1 to 2 minutes or until cooked through. Transfer to a plate and cover loosely with foil to keep warm. Repeat with remaining batter and blueberries. Dust with icing sugar and sprinkle with remaining blueberries. May be served with cream and maple syrup.

Serves 6 • • See recipe hints p.132

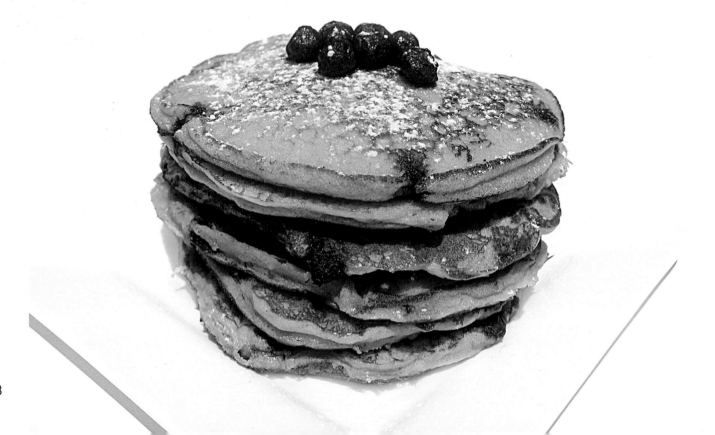

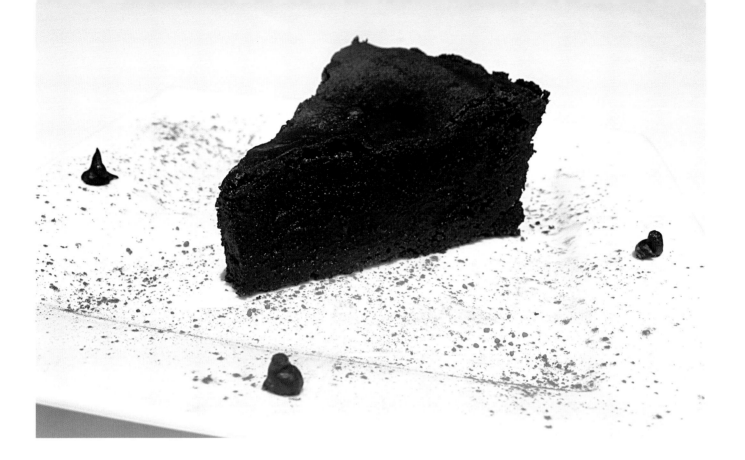

CHOCOLATE TART

1 x 200g pkt gluten free plain chocolate biscuits, crushed
80g butter, melted
250g good quality dark chocolate
150g butter, extra, at room temperature, cubed
3/4 cup (165g) caster sugar
2 tsp vanilla essence
1/4 cup (65ml) coffee liqueur (e.g. Kahlua, Tia Maria)
5 large eggs, at room temperature
2 Tbsp cocoa, for dusting

Pre-heat oven to 150°C. Grease 23cm fluted tart tin with cooking spray. Combine crushed chocolate biscuits and melted butter in a medium bowl. Mix until well combined. Press into the base and edges of tin, then place in the refrigerator.

Melt chocolate in a small bowl set over a small saucepan of boiling water. In a medium mixing bowl, beat butter, sugar, vanilla, coffee liqueur and one egg with electric beater until creamy. Add melted chocolate. Continue to beat until well combined. Clean beaters. In a large mixing bowl, beat four remaining eggs for 3 to 5 minutes, or until mixture has tripled in volume. Pour chocolate mixture into eggs, beat with electric beater for 1 to 2 minutes or until well combined, then pour into prepared base. Bake in pre-heated oven for 45 to 50 minutes or until set. Allow to cool on bench, then refrigerate for 2 to 3 hours. Serve with dusted cocoa and/or chocolate garnish.

Hint: If gluten free chocolate biscuits are unavailable, this tart can be made without base. Bake in 19cm springform tin instead.

Serves 12

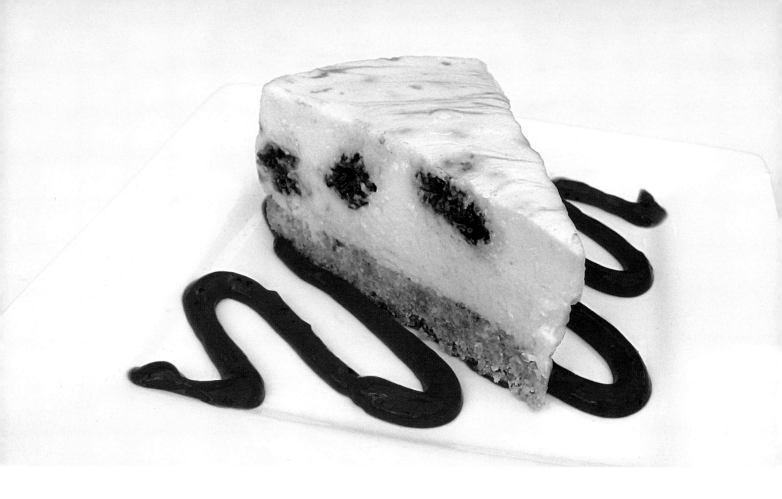

BLACKBERRY WHITE CHOCOLATE CHEESECAKE

1 x 200g pkt plain gluten free sweet biscuits
60g butter, melted
410g canned blackberries, reserve 1 Tbsp liquid
1/2 cup (125ml) boiling water
1 Tbsp gelatine
150g white chocolate buttons
500g reduced fat cream cheese
1 x 400g sweetened condensed skim milk
2 tsp vanilla essence

Crush biscuits to form fine crumbs. Add melted butter, mix until well combined. Press evenly into the base of a 19cm springform tin. Scatter tinned blackberries over base, ensuring evenly covered. Set aside.

Combine boiling water and gelatine in a small heat-proof bowl. Set bowl over larger bowl of boiling water, stirring constantly until all gelatine dissolved. Melt white chocolate buttons in a bowl set over a small saucepan of simmering water. Stir to ensure fully melted. In food processor, combine cream cheese, sweetened condensed milk, vanilla essence, dissolved gelatine and melted chocolate. Blend until well combined and even in consistency, then pour filling mixture over prepared base. Splash drops of reserved liquid on top of cheesecake. Run a knife or skewer in a straight motion up and down through drops, to form streaks on top of the cheesecake. Refrigerate for 3 to 4 hours or until set.

Hint: If lactose intolerant, this dessert is unsuitable. Half-serves may be tolerated.

Serves 10

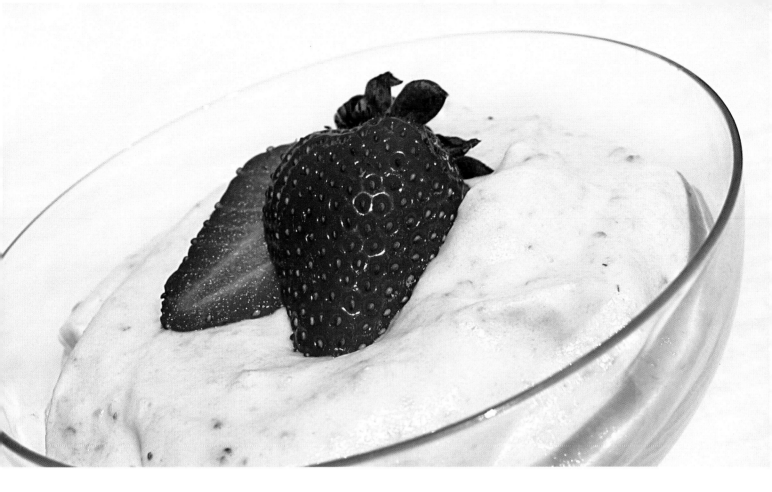

STRAWBERRY MOUSSE

1 Tbsp gelatine
1¹/2 Tbsp boiling water
500g strawberries, washed and hulled
3 Tbsp gluten free strawberry topping
1/4 cup (65ml) strawberry liqueur (optional)
1 cup (250ml) thickened cream
1/2 cup (110g) caster sugar
2 egg whites, at room temperature
6 fresh strawberries, cut in half

Combine boiling water and gelatine in a small heat-proof bowl. Set bowl over larger bowl of boiling water, stirring constantly until all gelatine dissolved. In a food processor, blend strawberries, strawberry topping and liqueur and dissolved gelatine until smooth in texture. Use 1 tsp gelatine, extra, if using liqueur. Set aside.

In a medium mixing bowl, whip cream with electric beaters until stiff peaks form. Fold strawberry mixture into whipped cream. In a clean bowl, beat egg whites until soft peaks form (eggs should triple in volume). Gradually beat in sugar until stiff peaks form. Fold beaten eggs through strawberry cream gently. Spoon evenly into six dessert dishes. Refrigerate for 1 to 2 hours or until set. Serve topped with a fresh strawberry.

Serves 6

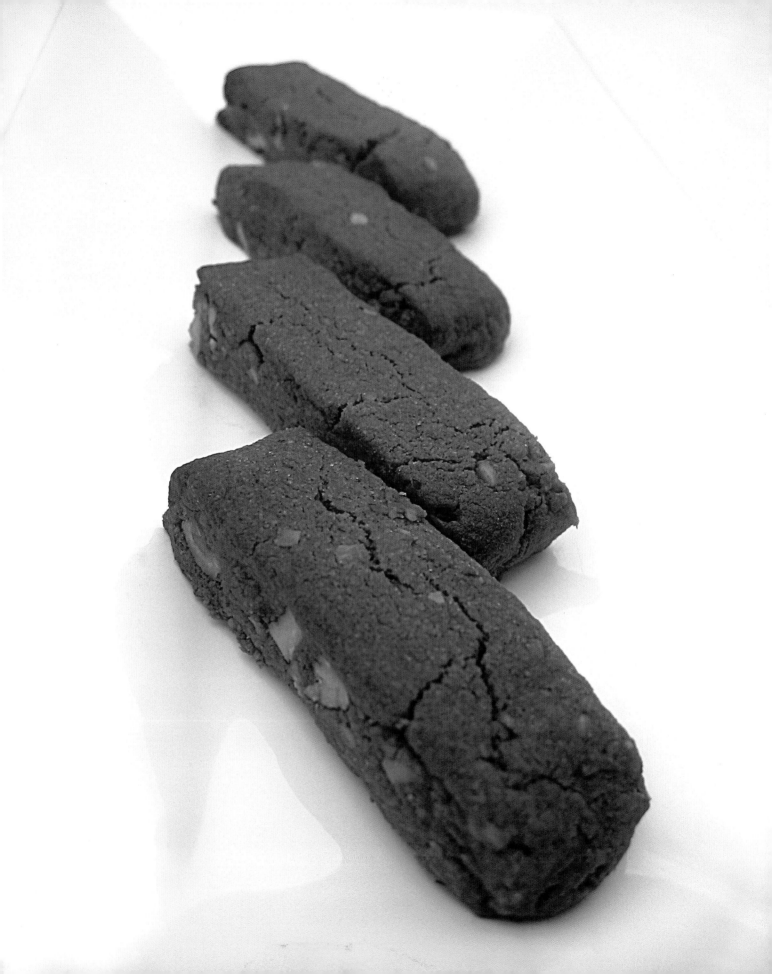

baked

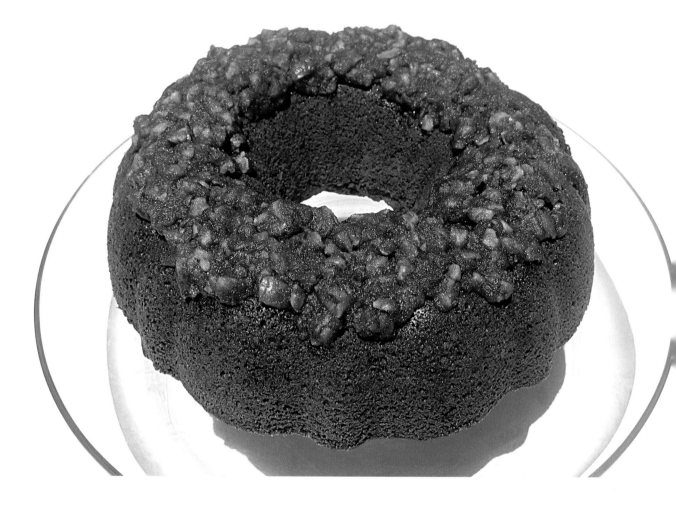

COFFEE CAKE

120g butter
3/4 cup (165g) sugar
1 tsp vanilla essence
3 eggs
2 Tbsp instant coffee, dissolved in 2 Tbsp hot water
1 cup (170g) rice flour
1/2 cup (80g) gluten free cornflour
1/2 cup (80g) potato flour •
1 tsp bicarb soda
2 tsp gluten free baking powder
1 tsp xanthan gum (optional) •
1 cup (250g) sour cream

Filling
80g butter, cubed at room temperature
3/4 cup (180g) firmly packed brown sugar
1 tsp ground cinnamon
1 Tbsp instant coffee powder
1 cup (125g) pecans, roughly chopped

Pre-heat oven to 180°C. Grease a ring cake pan. Cream butter, sugar and vanilla together in a large bowl with electric beaters. Add eggs, one at a time, beating well after each addition. Beat in dissolved coffee. Sift together flours, bicarb soda, baking powder and xanthan gum three times into a medium-sized bowl. Add to egg mixture, alternating with sour cream. Spread half of batter into greased ring pan. Spoon half of prepared filling on top of the cake batter, keeping within the centre portion of cake mix, careful not to touch sides of pan. Top with remaining half of cake batter. Bake in pre-heated oven for 30 to 35 minutes, or when firm to touch. When cooled, remove from pan and top with remaining filling.

Filling: Cream butter, brown sugar, cinnamon and instant coffee. Add chopped pecans, mix well.

• See recipe hints p.132

CARROT CAKE

1/3 cup (55g) rice flour
1/3 cup (50g) gluten free cornflour
2 tsp gluten free baking powder
1 tsp bicarb soda
1 tsp xanthan gum (optional) •
1 Tbsp ground cinnamon
1 Tbsp mixed spice
2 cups (200g) almond meal
1 cup (220g) brown sugar, firmly packed
2 medium (280g) carrots, grated
1/3 cup (40g) walnuts, chopped
4 eggs, separated

Cream Cheese Frosting
250g reduced fat cream cheese
1 Tbsp lemon juice
1/2 cup (85g) pure icing sugar
1/3 cup (40g) walnuts, chopped, extra

Pre-heat oven to 160°C. Grease a 22cm loaf pan and line with greaseproof baking paper. Sift flours, baking powder, bicarb soda, xanthan gum, cinnamon and mixed spice three times into a large mixing bowl. Stir in almond meal, sugar, carrot, walnuts and egg yolks. In a medium mixing bowl, beat egg whites until stiff peaks are formed. Gently fold egg whites into carrot mixture with a large metal spoon until just blended. Pour cake batter into prepared pan and bake in pre-heated oven for 45 to 50 minutes or until firm to touch (a skewer inserted into the centre should come out clean). Allow to stand for 10 minutes then remove from pan and place on wire rack to cool. When cool, top with cream cheese frosting and extra chopped walnuts.

Cream Cheese Frosting: Combine cream cheese, juice and icing sugar in a bowl. Mix well.

• See recipe hints p.132

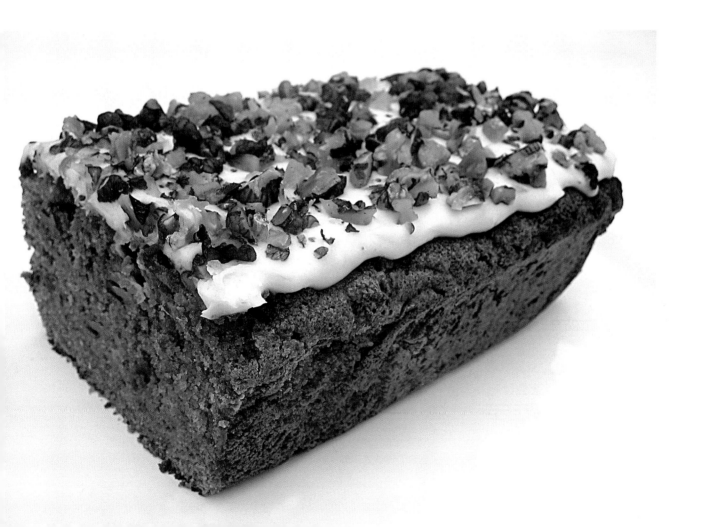

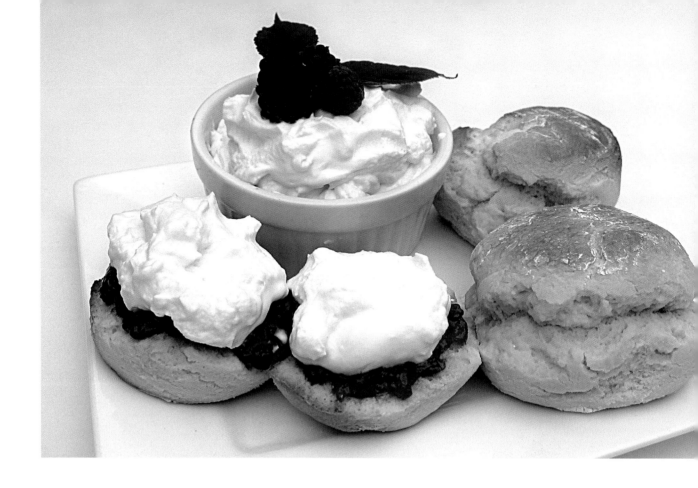

SCONES

150ml reduced fat milk •
1 egg
1 cup (170g) gluten free cornflour
1 cup (125g) tapioca flour •
1/2 cup (45g) soy flour •
1 tsp xanthan gum (optional) •
13/4 tsp gluten free baking powder
3 Tbsp caster sugar
80g butter, cubed, room temperature
2 Tbsp milk, extra •

Pre-heat oven to 200°C. Grease and flour a baking tray. Beat milk and egg together in a small bowl. Sift flours, xanthan gum, baking powder and sugar three times into a medium bowl. Rub in butter with fingertips until the mixture resembles fine breadcrumbs. Add the milk and egg mix all at once. Use a metal spoon to mix together until the mixture begins to hold together Then bring dough together with your hands. Turn the dough onto a lightly floured surface and knead gently about 4 to 5 times with your hands by pressing and then turning, until the dough is just smooth. Use a lightly floured rolling pin to roll out the dough until about 21/2 cm thick. Use a scone-cutter to cut out the scones, using a straight-down motion. Dip the cutter into cornflour before cutting out each scone. Place scones on prepared baking tray about 1cm apart. Brush the top of each scone with a little milk and bake in pre-heated oven for 10 to 12 minutes or until golden and cooked through. Remove the scones from the oven and immediately wrap them in a clean tea towel (this will help give them a soft crust). Serve warm with jam and whipped cream.

Flavour variations:
Cheese scones: omit sugar, add 1/2 cup grated tasty cheese and 1/4 tsp nutmeg after adding the milk
Cheese and herb: omit sugar, add 1/2 cup grated tasty cheese and 1 tsp mixed Italian herbs after adding the milk

Makes 12 •• See recipe hints p.132

CARAMEL NUT SLICE

1/2 cup (65g) fine rice flour •
1/4 cup (45g) potato flour •
1/3 cup (50g) gluten free cornflour
1/4 cup (75g) caster sugar
1/4 tsp bicarb soda
1/4 tsp gluten free baking powder
1 tsp xanthan gum (optional) •
60g butter, cubed, at room temperature
1 egg, beaten
1 tsp vanilla essence

Nut topping
1 cup (220g) brown sugar, firmly packed
150g butter, cubed, at room temperature
1/3 cup (85ml) cream
2 1/2 Tbsp gluten free cornflour
1/2 cup (65g) pecan nuts, roughly chopped
2/3 cup (110g) Brazil nuts, roughly chopped
1/2 cup (75g) macadamia nuts, cut in half

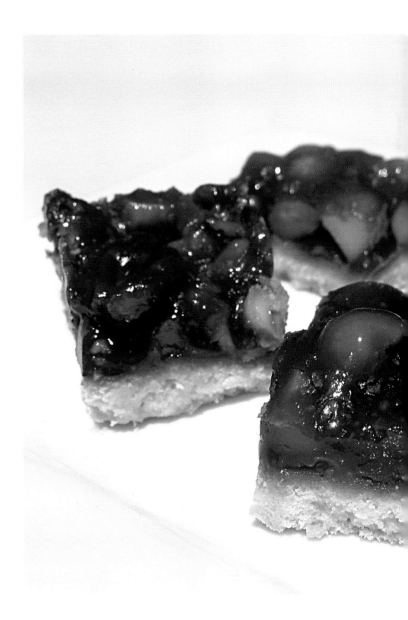

Pre-heat oven to 180°C. Grease a 27cm x 17cm shallow baking tray, and line with greaseproof paper.
Sift flours, sugar, bicarb soda, baking powder and xanthan gum three times into a bowl. Add melted butter, beaten egg and vanilla essence, mixing until well combined. As mixture becomes more solid, use your hands to bring together to form a ball. Roll pastry to 5mm thickness between two sheets of baking paper. Place into lined pan. Use a fork to prick the pastry all over. Cover and place in the refrigerator for 10 minutes, then bake in pre-heated oven for 10 to 12 minutes, until base is light golden brown. Set aside to cool.

Spread prepared nut topping over base and bake in pre-heated oven for 15 to 20 minutes. Leave on bench to cool, then refrigerate for 3 hours before cutting into squares.

Nut topping: Place sugar and butter in a large saucepan. Cook over medium heat, stirring constantly, until butter melts and mixture comes to the boil. Remove from heat, stir in cream and cornflour, mixing until smooth. Add pecan, Brazil and macadamia nuts, mix well. Return saucepan to medium heat and stir until mixture comes to the boil. Turn down heat to low, and cook for further 2 to 3 minutes.

Makes 30   • See recipe hints p.132

LEMON LIME CHIFFON CAKE

3/4 cup (130g) rice flour
1/2 cup (70g) soy flour •
1/2 cup (80g) gluten free cornflour
1 1/4 cups (270g) caster sugar
1 tsp xanthan gum (optional) •
2 tsp gluten free baking powder
4 large eggs, separated
1/2 cup (125ml) canola oil
1/2 cup (125ml) lemon juice
2 Tbsp (40ml) lime juice
1 tsp lemon rind, finely grated
1 tsp lime rind, finely grated
1 tsp vanilla essence
1/4 tsp cream of tartar

Pre-heat oven to 160°C. Grease a deep ring pan. Sift flours, sugar, baking powder and xanthan gum three times into a large mixing bowl. Make a well in the centre of the flour. Add egg yolks, oil, lemon and lime juice, rind and vanilla. Beat with electric beaters until well combined. In a medium mixing bowl, beat egg whites with cream of tartar until soft peaks form. With a metal spoon, fold half of the beaten egg whites at a time into the flour mixture. Ensure well combined. Pour mixture into prepared tin, bake 30 to 35 minutes, or until firm to touch (a skewer inserted into the centre should come out clean). Invert the cake onto a wire rack, but leave to cool completely in the tin, approximately 3 to 4 hours. Remove cake from tin only once cool.

• See recipe hints p.132

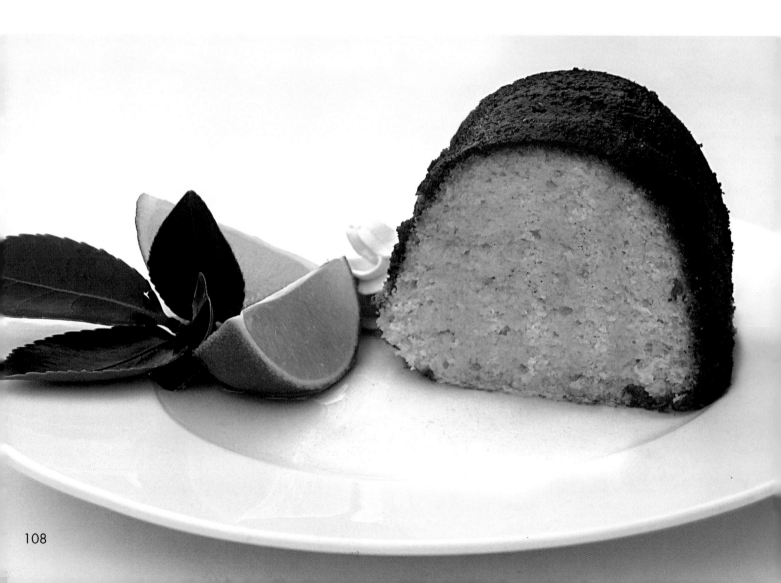

HAZELNUT CRESCENTS

1/3 cup (55g) rice flour
1/4 cup (35g) gluten free cornflour
1/4 cup (55g) sugar
11/4 cups (125g) hazelnut meal
100g unsalted butter, cubed
1 egg yolk, whisked, room temperature
1 tsp vanilla essence
1/2 cup (85g) pure icing sugar, to dust

Pre-heat oven to 160°C. Grease two baking trays. Sift flours into a medium mixing bowl. Add sugar and hazelnut meal. Rub in butter. Mix in egg yolk and vanilla essence with a metal spoon, then use your hands to bring the mixture together to form a dough. Turn onto a cornfloured board and knead lightly. Divide into two even portions and wrap in plastic wrap and refrigerate for 15 minutes. Remove biscuit dough from refrigerator, roll into a log approximately 2cm thick. Cut every 11/2 to 2cm, and shape into a rounded crescent shape. Place formed biscuit dough on prepared baking tray, bake in pre-heated oven for 15 to 20 minutes or until lightly browned. Remove from oven, leave to cool on trays for 5 minutes. Roll in icing sugar then transfer to wire rack to cool completely. Dust with additional icing sugar prior to serving.

Makes 30

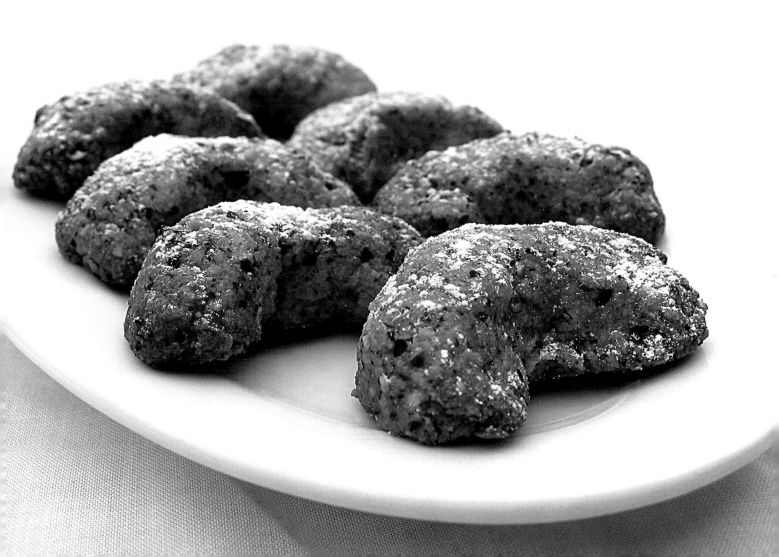

TASTY HIGH FIBRE MUFFINS

1 cup (170g) brown rice flour
1/2 cup (75g) gluten free cornflour
1/2 cup (45g) soy flour •
2 tsp gluten free baking powder
1 tsp bicarb soda
1 tsp xanthan gum (optional) •
3 eggs
80g butter, melted
1/2 cup (125ml) water
200g gluten free natural yoghurt
1 cup (120g) parmesan cheese, grated
1/2 medium (75g) zucchini, grated
1/2 cup (80g) sunflower kernels
1/2 cup (60g) rice bran
1/4 cup (30g) walnuts, crushed
1/4 tsp ground nutmeg

Pre-heat oven to 170°C. Grease a 12 muffin pan tray. Sift flours, baking powder, bicarb soda, and xanthan gum three times into a large mixing bowl. In a medium mixing bowl, mix eggs, melted butter, water, yoghurt, cheese, zucchini, sunflower seeds, rice bran, walnuts and nutmeg. Mix until well combined. Pour this mixture into the sifted flours. Beat well with wooden spoon for 2 to 3 minutes. Pour muffin mix into greased muffin pans, to 2/3 full. Bake in pre-heated oven for 12 to 15 minutes or until firm to touch (a skewer inserted into the centre should come out clean). Allow to stand for 5 minutes before removing from pans. Place on wire rack to cool.

Makes 12   • See recipe hints p.132

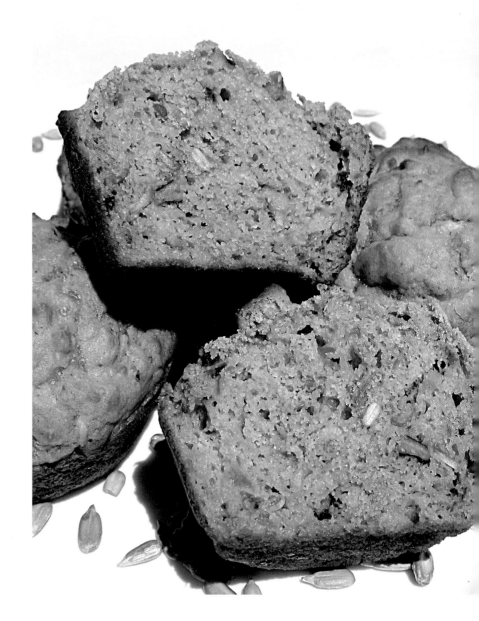

TOMATO AND SPINACH SAVOURY MUFFINS

1 cup (170g) rice flour
1/2 cup (75g) gluten free cornflour
1/2 cup (45g) soy flour •
2 tsp gluten free baking powder
1 tsp bicarb soda
1 tsp xanthan gum (optional) •
3 eggs
80g butter, melted
200g gluten free natural yoghurt
1 cup (250ml) reduced fat milk •
100g parmesan cheese, grated
2 medium (280g) tomatoes, diced
2 cups (70g) baby spinach leaves, roughly chopped
salt, freshly ground black pepper to taste

Pre-heat oven to 170°C. Grease a 12 muffin pan tray. Sift flours, baking powder, bicarb soda and xanthan gum three times into a large mixing bowl. In a medium mixing bowl, mix eggs, melted butter, yoghurt, milk, cheese, tomato and spinach. Season with salt and pepper. Stir until well combined. Pour this mixture into the sifted flours, mix well, beating well with wooden spoon for 2 to 3 minutes. Pour muffin mix into greased pans, until they are 2/3 full. Bake in pre-heated oven for 12 to 15 minutes or until firm to touch (a skewer inserted into the centre should come out clean). Allow to stand for 5 minutes. Remove from pans and place on wire rack to cool.

Makes 12 •• See recipe hints p.132

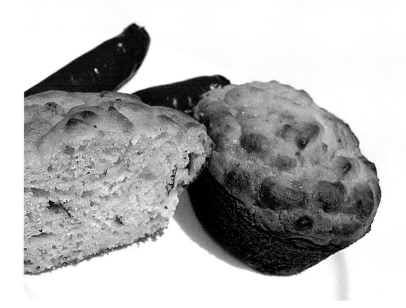

CHILLI CHEESE SAVOURY MUFFINS

1 cup (170g) rice flour
1/2 cup (75g) gluten free cornflour
1/2 cup (45g) soy flour •
2 tsp gluten free baking powder
1 tsp bicarb soda
1 tsp xanthan gum (optional) •
1 tsp chilli powder
3 eggs
80g butter, melted
200g gluten free natural yoghurt
3/4 cup (190ml) reduced fat milk •
3/4 cup (90g) parmesan cheese, grated
1 cup (100g) tasty cheese, grated
2 Tbsp parsley, finely chopped
salt, freshly ground black pepper to taste

Pre-heat oven to 170°C. Grease a 12 muffin pan tray. Sift flours, baking powder, bicarb soda, xanthan gum and chilli three times into a large mixing bowl. In a medium mixing bowl, mix eggs, melted butter, yoghurt, milk, cheeses and parsley. Season with salt and pepper. Stir until well combined. Pour this mixture into sifted flours. Beat with electric beaters for 2 to 3 minutes. Pour muffin mix into greased muffin pans, to 2/3 full. Bake in pre-heated oven for 12 to 15 minutes or until firm to touch (a skewer inserted into the centre should come out clean). Allow to stand for 5 minutes before removing from pans. Place on wire rack to cool.

Makes 12 •• See recipe hints p.132

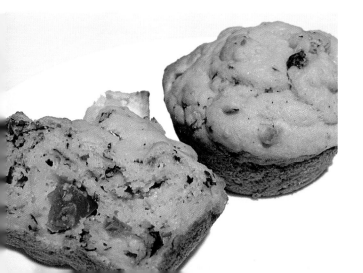

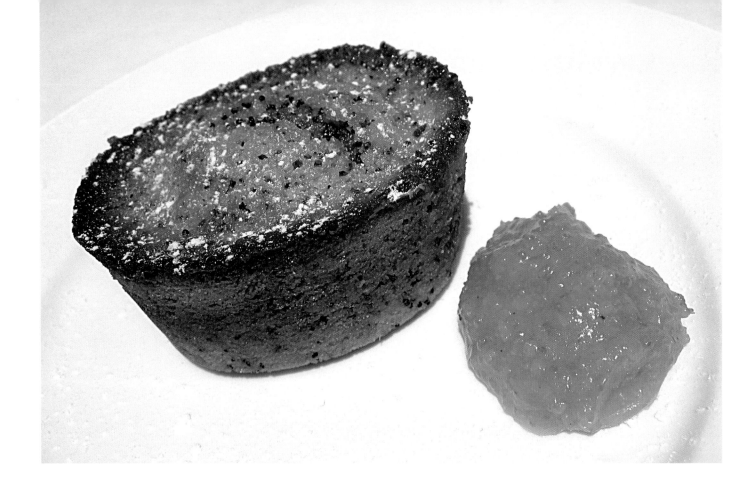

ORANGE POPPY SEED FRIANDS WITH ORANGE CURD

140g unsalted butter
2 cups (330g) pure icing sugar, plus extra to dust
1/4 (40g) gluten free cornflour
1/4 cup (45g) fine rice flour •
1 1/4 cups (125g) almond meal
1/3 cup (40g) poppy seeds
rind of one orange, finely grated
5 egg whites, lightly whisked
2 Tbsp orange juice
1 tsp vanilla essence

Orange curd
1 tsp orange rind, finely grated
juice from 1 orange
1 egg
1/3 cup (75g) caster sugar
40g unsalted butter
1/2 tsp gluten free cornflour

Pre-heat oven to 180°C. Lightly grease 12 friand pans (or petite loaf pans). Place butter in small saucepan over low heat. Once it has melted, cook for further 3 to 4 minutes until you start to see flecks of brown appear. Set aside.

Sift icing sugar and flours three times into a bowl. Mix in almond meal, poppy seeds and orange rind, combining well. Add egg whites, vanilla essence, orange juice and butter to dry ingredients. Use a metal spoon to combine. Spoon mixture into prepared pans, until they are 2/3 full. Bake in pre-heated oven for 12 to 15 minutes until light golden and firm to touch. Allow to stand for 5 minutes prior to removing from tins, then place on wire rack to cool. Dust with pure icing sugar and orange curd.

Orange Curd: Place rind, juice, egg, sugar, butter and cornflour in a small heavy-based saucepan and stir to combine. Cook over low heat, stirring constantly for 10 minutes or until thick. Pour into a small bowl. Cover and refrigerate to set.

Makes 12   • See recipe hints p.132

PUMPKIN SPICE MUFFINS

1 cup (170g) rice flour
1/2 cup (75g) gluten free cornflour
1/2 cup (90g) potato flour •
1 tsp bicarb soda
2 tsp gluten free baking powder
1 tsp xanthan gum (optional) •
2 Tbsp mixed spice
1 Tbsp ground cinnamon
40g butter, melted
200g gluten free vanilla yoghurt
2 eggs
1 1/2 cups (400g) pumpkin, cooked, mashed
1 cup (220g) sugar

Pre-heat oven to 170°C. Grease a deep, 12 muffin pan tray. Sift flours, bicarb soda, baking powder, xanthan gum and spices three times into a large bowl. In a medium mixing bowl, combine melted butter, yoghurt and eggs. Stir in cooled pumpkin and sugar. Add this mixture into sifted flours, then mix well with electric beater for 2 to 3 minutes. Pour muffin mix into 12 greased muffin pans, to 2/3 full. Cook for 12 to 15 minutes or until golden brown and skewer comes out clean when inserted into the centre of the muffin.

Makes 12   • See recipe hints p.132

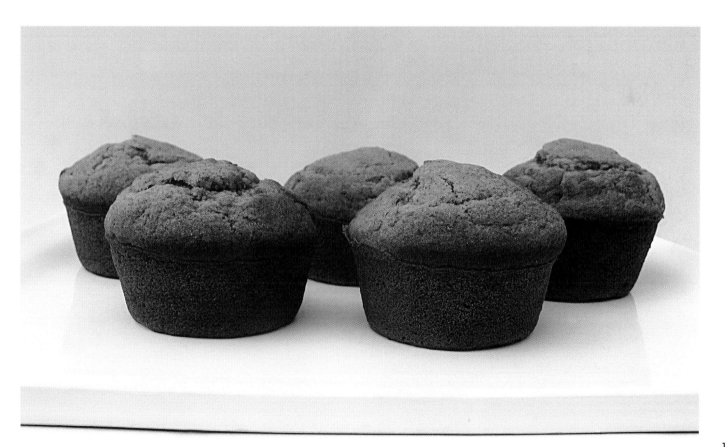

PEANUT BUTTER AND SESAME BISCUITS

30g butter
1 cup (300g) peanut butter
3 Tbsp brown sugar
2 Tbsp caster sugar
2 eggs, lightly beaten
1 tsp vanilla essence
3 Tbsp sesame seeds
2/3 cup (85g) fine rice flour •
2/3 cup (95g) gluten free cornflour
1/2 cup (40g) soy flour •
1/2 tsp bicarb soda
1 tsp xanthan gum (optional) •

Pre-heat oven to 180°C. Grease two baking trays.
In a mixing bowl, cream butter, peanut butter and sugars
with electric beaters. Add eggs, vanilla essence and
sesame seeds, beat well. Sift flours, bicarb soda and
xanthan gum three times. Add sifted flours to peanut
butter mixture, mix until well combined. Shape into balls
then flatten to 5mm thick. Place onto tray and bake in
oven for 10 to 12 minutes or until golden brown.
Remove from oven, leave to cool on trays for 5 minutes
then transfer to wire rack to cool completely.

Makes 40   • See recipe hints p.132

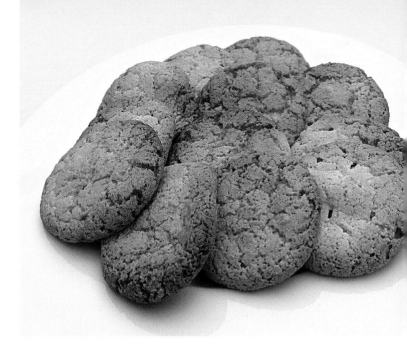

ALMOND BISCUITS

3/4 cup (75g) almond meal
1 Tbsp gluten free cornflour
1/2 tsp gluten free baking powder
1 egg white
1/2 cup (110g) caster sugar
1 tsp lemon rind, finely grated
3 drops almond essence
1 Tbsp butter, melted

Pre-heat oven to 140°C. Line two baking trays with non-stick
baking paper. In a small bowl, combine almond meal,
cornflour, and baking powder. In a separate bowl, beat egg
whites with electric beaters until firm. Gradually beat in the
sugar, continue beating for 5 minutes or until stiff peaks form.
Beat in ground almond mix, lemon rind, almond essence and
melted butter with a metal spoon. Roll 2 teaspoons of biscuit
mixture into balls. Flatten slightly, place on prepared baking
trays. Bake in pre-heated oven for 25 minutes. Remove from
oven, leave to cool on trays for 5 minutes then transfer to wire
rack to cool completely.

Makes 40

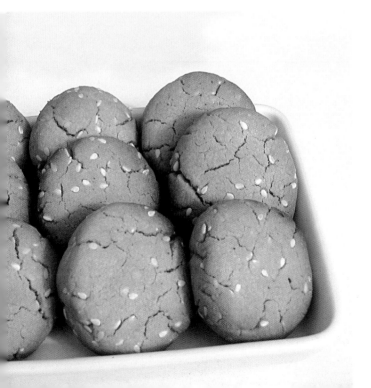

MICROWAVE FUDGE-CARAMEL

1 x 400g can sweetened condensed milk
100g butter, cubed
1 cup (220g) firmly packed brown sugar

Line a 20cm square pan with greaseproof paper. Place sweetened condensed milk, butter and brown sugar into a deep three-litre microwave-proof container. Cook on medium-high setting for total of 10 to 12 minutes. (Mixture will bubble up, carefully stir down every 2 minutes or more often as required). Finally, add flavour of choice while mixture is still boiling hot, stirring until well combined. Pour into the prepared pan, then place in the refrigerator for 4 to 6 hours or until firm. Remove from refrigerator and cut into 2cm x 2cm pieces.

Suggested flavours:
Irish cream: 1/4 cup Irish cream liqueur
Peppermint: 1/4 tsp peppermint essence (more to taste) and 2 Tbsp cream
Vanilla: 1 Tbsp vanilla essence and 2 Tbsp cream

Hint: If lactose intolerant, limit intake to one piece. Recipe has been developed for 1000W microwave. Cooking times and settings may need to be adjusted for different microwaves. Refer to user guide.

Makes 30 pieces

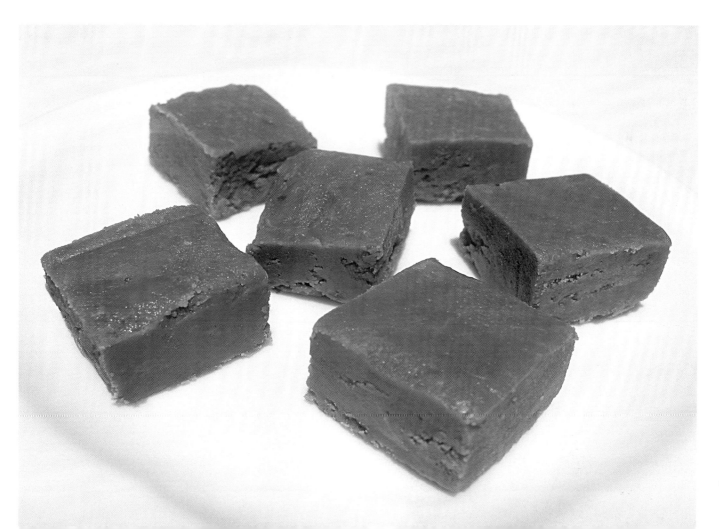

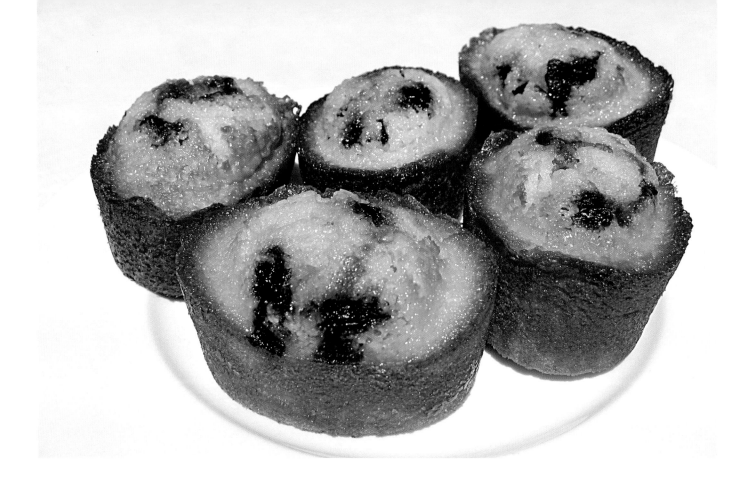

BERRY FRIANDS

140g unsalted butter
2 cups (330g) pure icing sugar, plus extra to dust
1/4 cup (40g) gluten free cornflour
1/4 cup (45g) rice flour
1 1/4 cups (125g) almond meal
5 egg whites, lightly whisked
1 Tbsp lemon juice
2 tsp vanilla essence
150g blueberries, boysenberries, or raspberries

Pre-heat oven to 180°C. Lightly grease 12 friand pans. Melt butter in a small saucepan over low heat. Heat for further 3 to 4 minutes until flecks of brown appear. Set aside. Sift icing sugar and flours three times into a bowl. Mix in almond meal, combining well. Add egg whites, lemon juice, vanilla and butter to dry ingredients. Use a metal spoon to combine. Spoon mixture into prepared pans, until they are 2/3 full. Add berries, centred on top of batter. Bake in pre-heated oven for 12 to 15 minutes until light golden and firm to touch (a skewer inserted into the centre should come out clean). Allow to stand for 5 minutes before removing from tins, then place on wire rack to cool. Dust with pure icing sugar when serving.

Makes 12

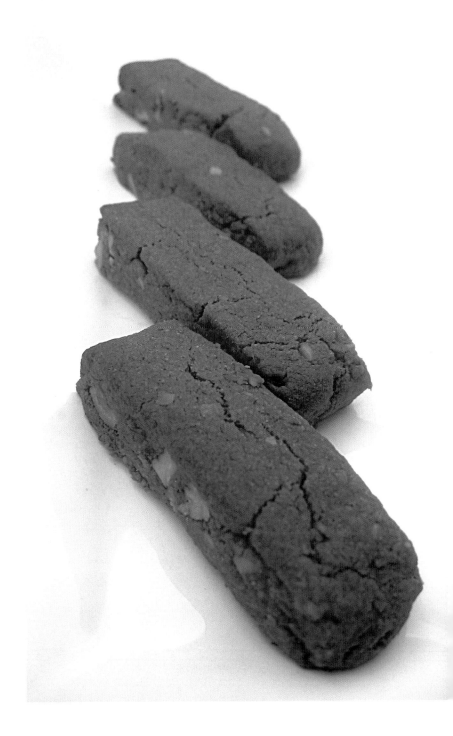

CHOCOLATE PECAN SHORTBREAD

1/2 cup (85g) pure icing sugar
2/3 cup (85g) fine rice flour •
1/2 cup (45g) soy flour •
3/4 cup (110g) gluten free corn flour
1 tsp xanthan gum (optional) •
2 Tbsp cocoa
150g butter, cubed, at room temperature
1/2 cup (65g) pecan nuts, finely chopped

Pre-heat oven to 140°C. Grease baking trays with cooking spray. Sift icing sugar, flours, xanthan gum and cocoa together three times into a bowl.
Rub in butter with fingertips until it resembles fine breadcrumbs. Add chopped pecans. Work dough together with your hands to form a ball. This will take some time. Once a kneadable dough is obtained, roll between two sheets of baking paper, to 1 1/2 cm thickness. Cut 2cm x 5cm fingers of shortbread. Place on prepared baking trays and bake in pre-heated oven for 30 minutes or until cooked. Remove from oven and cool on tray for 5 minutes, before transferring to a wire rack to cool completely.

Makes 15   • See recipe hints p.132

MOIST CHOCOLATE CAKE WITH JAFFA ICING

1 cup (170g) rice flour
1/2 cup (75g) gluten free cornflour
1/2 cup (90g) potato flour •
2/3 cup (70g) cocoa
2 tsp gluten free baking powder
1 tsp bicarb soda
1 tsp xanthan gum (optional) •
2 eggs
11/2 cups (330g) sugar
50g butter, melted
200g gluten free vanilla yoghurt
2/3 cup (165ml) reduced fat milk •
1 tsp vanilla essence

Pre-heat oven to 170°C. Grease a 23cm springform cake pan. Sift flours, cocoa, baking powder, bicarb soda, and xanthan gum three times into a large mixing bowl. In a medium mixing bowl, mix eggs and sugar until thick and foamy. Add melted butter, yoghurt, milk and vanilla essence into egg mixture, stir until well combined. Pour this mixture into sifted flours. Beat with electric beaters for 2 to 3 minutes. Pour cake batter into greased pan and bake in pre-heated oven for 30 to 35 minutes or until firm to touch (a skewer inserted into the centre should come out clean). Allow to stand for 5 minutes. Remove from pan and place on wire rack to cool. Top with jaffa icing.

Ideas for icing:

Jaffa chocolate ganache: melt 200g chocolate, stir in 3 Tbsp cream, 2 tsp grated orange rind. Remove from heat, allow to cool before icing cake.
Jaffa butter cream icing: combine 100g unsalted butter, 2 cups (220g) pure icing sugar, 3 Tbsp orange juice, 3 tsp orange rind, 2 Tbsp cocoa powder.

• • See recipe hints p.132.

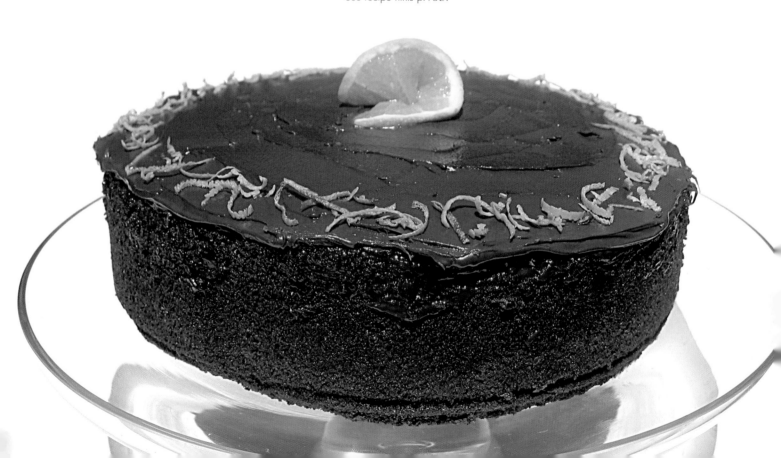

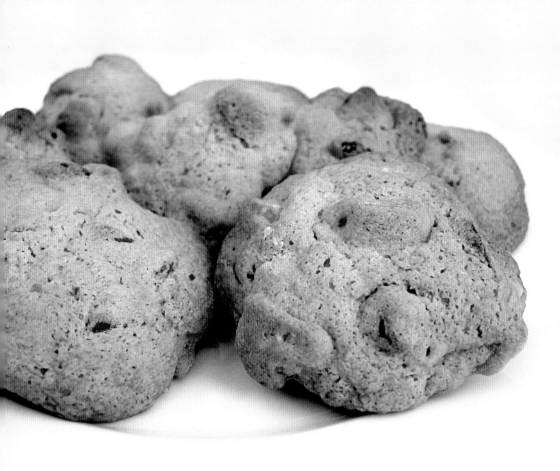

MACADAMIA CHOC CHIP COOKIES

125g unsalted butter
1/4 cup (40g) brown sugar
1/4 cup (55g) caster sugar
1 egg
1 tsp vanilla essence
2/3 cup (110g) rice flour
1/2 cup (75g) gluten free cornflour
1/4 cup (20g) soy flour •
1/2 tsp bicarb soda
100g chocolate chips
1/2 cup (75g) macadamia nuts

Pre-heat oven to 170°C. Grease two baking trays. In a medium mixing bowl, cream butter and sugars with electric beaters. Add egg and vanilla essence, beat well.

Sift flours and bicarb soda three times into a bowl. Add to egg mixture, beat well. Add chocolate chips and macadamia nuts, stir with wooden spoon until well combined. Place spoonfuls onto prepared tray. Bake in pre-heated oven for 8 to 10 minutes or until golden brown. Remove from oven, leave to cool on trays for 5 minutes then transfer to wire rack to cool completely.

Flavour variation:
Ginger and Brazil nut: substitute chocolate and macadamia nuts with 2 tsp ground ginger, 60g crystallised ginger, finely chopped, 1/2 cup (85g) brazil nuts, chopped

Makes 20   • See recipe hints p.132

119

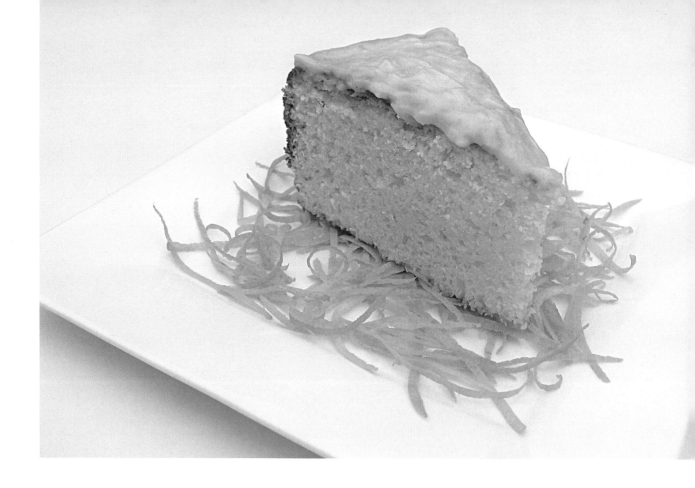

LEMON RICOTTA CAKE

1 cup (170g) rice flour
1/2 cup (75g) gluten free cornflour
1/2 cup (90g) potato flour •
2 tsp gluten free baking powder
1 tsp bicarb soda
1 tsp xanthan gum (optional) •
2 eggs
11/2 cups (330g) sugar
60g butter, melted
3/4 cup (200g) ricotta cheese
rind of one lemon, finely grated
3/4 cup (190ml) lemon juice

Lemon Ricotta Icing
2/3 cup (175g) ricotta cheese
1/3 cup (55g) pure icing sugar
1 tsp lemon rind, finely grated

Pre-heat oven to 170°C. Grease a 23cm springform cake pan. Sift flours, baking powder, bicarb soda, and xanthan gum three times into a large mixing bowl. In a medium mixing bowl, mix eggs and sugar until thick and foamy. Add melted butter, ricotta cheese, lemon rind and juice into egg mixture, stir until well combined. Pour this mixture into sifted flours. Beat with electric beaters for 2 to 3 minutes. Pour cake batter into greased pan, bake in pre-heated oven for 30 to 35 minutes or until firm to touch (a skewer inserted into the centre should come out clean). Allow to stand for 5 minutes. Remove from pan and place on wire rack to cool. Top with lemon ricotta icing when cool.

Lemon Ricotta Icing: In a small bowl, mix ricotta cheese, icing sugar and lemon rind together until well combined.

• See recipe hints p.132

BANANA CHOC CHIP MUFFINS

1 cup (170g) rice flour
1/2 cup (75g) gluten free cornflour
1/2 cup (45g) soy flour •
2 tsp gluten free baking powder
1 tsp bicarb soda
1 tsp xanthan gum (optional) •
2 eggs
1 cup (220g) caster sugar
50g butter, melted
1 tsp vanilla essence
2 medium (260g) bananas, mashed
1/3 cup (85ml) milk
200g gluten free vanilla yoghurt
180g chocolate chips

Pre-heat oven to 170°C. Grease a 12 muffin pan tray (or use patty pans). Sift flours, baking powder, bicarb soda, and xanthan gum three times into a large mixing bowl. In a medium mixing bowl, beat eggs and sugar with electric beaters until thick and foamy. Add melted butter, vanilla essence, banana, milk, yoghurt, into egg mixture, beat until well combined. Pour this mixture into sifted flours. Beat for further 2 to 3 minutes. Finally, add choc chips, stir through with a metal spoon until well combined. Pour muffin batter into muffin pans, to 2/3 full. Bake in pre-heated oven for 12 to 15 minutes or until firm to touch (a skewer inserted into the centre should come out clean). Allow to stand for 5 minutes. Remove from pans and place on wire rack to cool.

Makes 12   • See recipe hints p.132

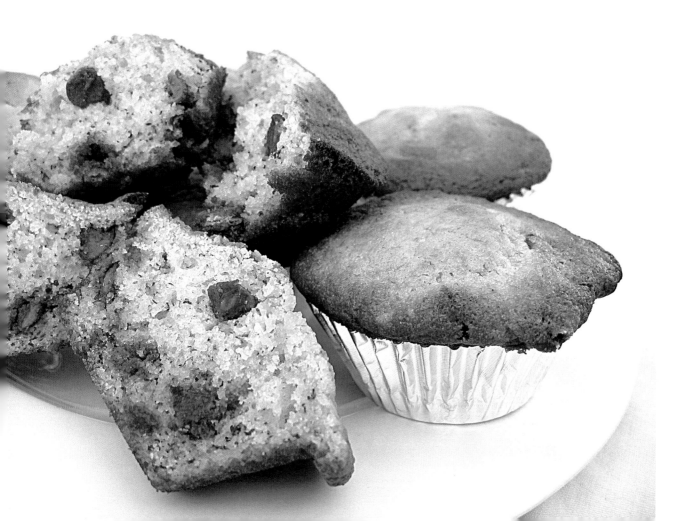

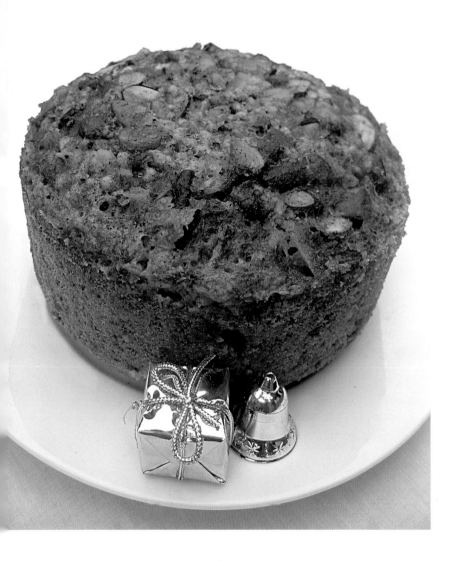

NUTTY CHRISTMAS PUD

100g Brazil nuts, roughly chopped
100g pecan nuts, roughly chopped
250g almonds, roughly chopped
50g macadamia nuts, roughly chopped
1/2 cup (125ml) brandy
100g butter
1/2 cup (110g) brown sugar, firmly packed
1/2 cup (85g) rice flour
1/4 cup (45g) potato flour •
1/4 cup (35g) gluten free cornflour
1/2 cup (110g) brown sugar, firmly packed, extra
2 tsp mixed spice
1 tsp ground cinnamon
1/4 tsp ground nutmeg
1/4 tsp ground cloves
3/4 cup (85g) fresh gluten free breadcrumbs
2 eggs, lightly beaten
1/4 cup (65ml) milk

Place all nuts in medium bowl, pour over with brandy. Toss to combine well. Cover, and place in the refrigerator to soak overnight.

Grease 15cm steamed pudding basin. Line base with greaseproof paper. In a medium saucepan, combine soaked nuts, butter and 1/2 cup of brown sugar. Stir over medium heat until butter has melted and sugar has dissolved and caramelised. Sift flours, extra brown sugar and spices three times into a large mixing bowl. Stir in gluten free breadcrumbs. Add caramelised nuts, eggs and milk to dry ingredients. Beat well with a wooden spoon. Pour into prepared pudding basin. Place pudding basin in large stockpot, fill with water to half-way up side of basin. Steam for 11/2 to 2 hours over medium-low heat.

Hint: Best if cooked on day of serving, however can be steamed early, and refrigerated until required. Re-heat on day of serving by steaming for 20 to 30 minutes.

• See recipe hints p.132

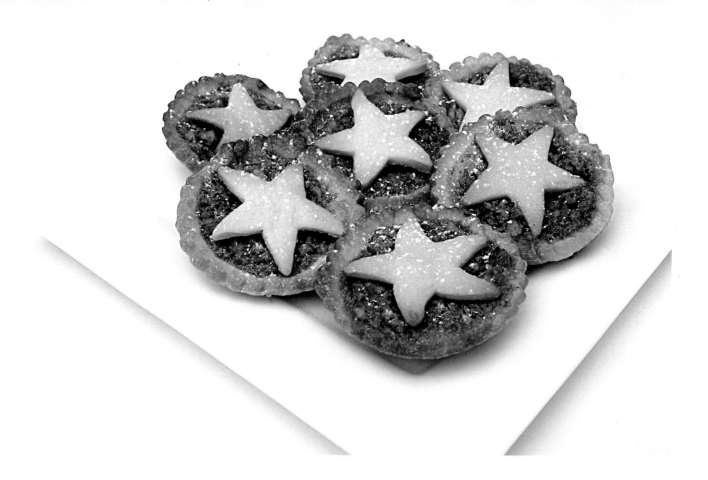

PECAN MINCE TARTS

Pastry
1/2 cup (65g) fine rice flour •
1/4 cup (35g) gluten free cornflour
1/4 cup (20g) soy flour •
1 tsp xanthan gum (optional) •
2 Tbsp caster sugar
80g butter
3 Tbsp (120ml) iced water

Filling
20g butter, unsalted
1/4 cup (55g) brown sugar, firmly packed
1/2 tsp vanilla essence
1 egg
1/4 cup (65ml) maple syrup
1/2 cup (65g) pecans, roughly chopped

Pre-heat oven to 170°C. Grease individual tartlet trays and one baking tray.

Pastry: Sift flours and xanthan gum three times into a bowl. Combine sifted flours, sugar and butter in food processor. Process until it resembles fine breadcrumbs. While the motor is running, add iced water (one tablespoon at a time) to allow mixture to form soft dough. Knead on gluten-free floured board. Wrap in plastic wrap and refrigerate for 30 minutes before rolling to use. Roll pastry 2mm thick between two sheets of greaseproof paper. Cut with scalloped pastry cutter to fit tartlet tray. Place pastry in tins, trim edges to neaten. Use a star-shaped pastry cutter to cut pastry stars. Place on flat baking tray. Bake cases and stars in pre-heated oven for 10 minutes or until golden brown (stars will only take 7 to 8 minutes). Leave oven on 170°C.

Filling: Cream butter, sugar and vanilla in a mixing bowl with electric beaters. Add egg and maple syrup, beat well. Finally stir in chopped pecans. Pour the filling into prepared pastry shells. Bake for 5 to 10 minutes or until the filling is set. (Centre should remain firm when given a gentle shake.) Place pastry star on tart while still warm. Let tarts stand for 10 minutes before removing from tins. Then transfer to wire rack to cool completely.

Makes 24 • See recipe hints p. 132

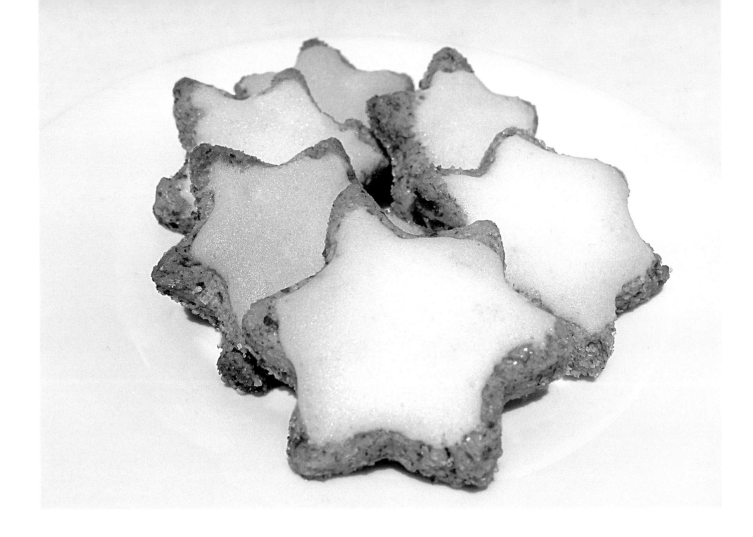

CHRISTMAS STAR BISCUITS

1 cup (100g) ground almonds
5 Tbsp (60g) gluten free cornflour
1 1/2 tsp ground cinnamon
1/2 tsp gluten free baking powder
1 egg white
1/2 cup (110g) caster sugar
1 Tbsp butter, melted

Icing
1/2 cup pure icing sugar
2 1/2 tsp lemon juice

Pre-heat oven to 140°C. Line two baking trays with grease-proof paper. In a small bowl, combine ground almonds, cornflour, cinnamon and baking powder. In a separate bowl, beat egg whites with electric beaters until soft peaks form. Gradually beat in the sugar until stiff peaks form.

With a metal spoon, mix in ground almond mixture and melted butter. Knead on a corn-floured board. Roll between two sheets of baking paper to approximately 3mm thick. Use star-shaped cookie cutter to cut biscuits. Place on prepared baking trays. Bake in pre-heated oven for 7 minutes, leave oven on. Remove from oven, leave to cool on trays for 2 minutes, spread neatly with prepared icing, then return to oven to bake for further 2 minutes. Remove from oven, leave to cool on trays for 5 minutes then transfer to wire rack to cool completely.

Icing: Combine icing sugar and lemon juice in a bowl.

Makes 50

CHOCOLATE TRUFFLES

1 x 200g packet gluten free plain sweet biscuits
1/3 cup (35g) cocoa
1/3 cup (115ml) sweetened condensed milk
11/2 Tbsp rum or brandy (adjust according
  to liking)
1 x 160g packet gluten free chocolate sprinkles

Crush gluten free biscuits to form crumbs.
Mix biscuit crumbs and cocoa in medium bowl
until well combined. Add condensed milk and
brandy, mixing with hands until a firm dough
is formed. Shape spoonfuls of mixture into balls,
toss in chocolate sprinkles to coat. Refrigerate
until firm.

Makes 25

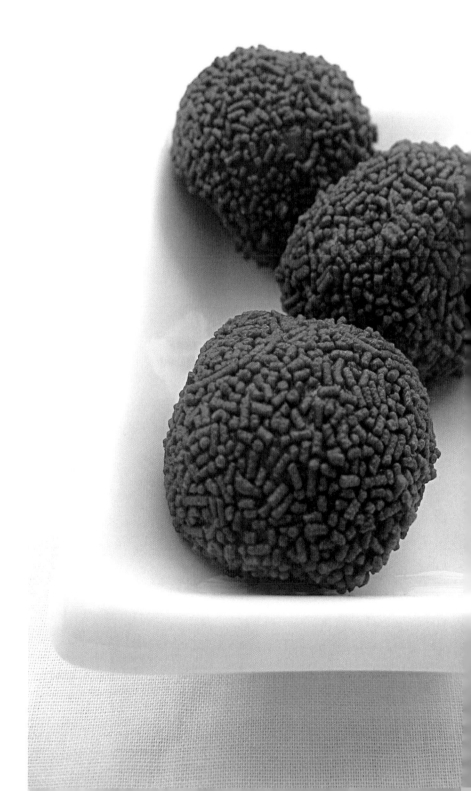

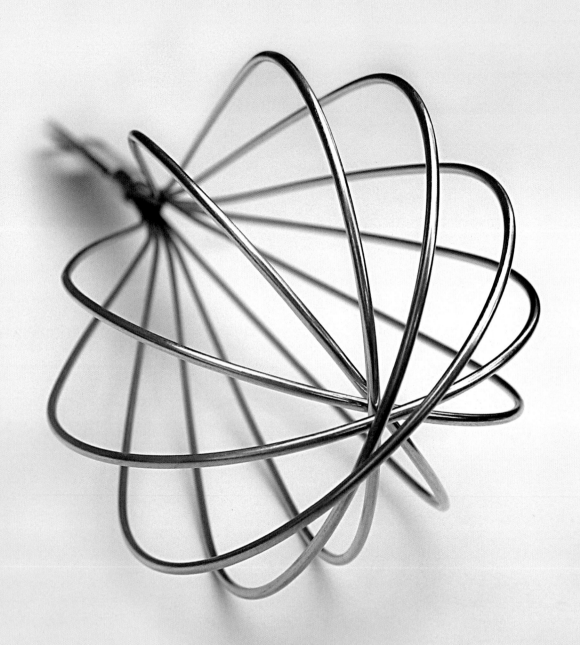

index

RECIPE HINTS

INGREDIENT SUBSTITUTIONS

• Lactose intolerance

Where recipes include milk or other lactose containing ingredients in large quantities, the following substitutions are recommended:
- replace regular milk with lactose-free milk
- substitute evaporated milk with 1/2 quantity lactose free milk and 1/2 quantity cream
- substitute yoghurt for lactose free yoghurt
- replace ice cream with lactose free ice cream

This is a guide only. Individual sensitivity may call for further recipe modification.

• Sorbitol intolerance

If stone fruits do not agree with you (perhaps due to sorbitol intolerance), substitute for alternative fruit; e.g. pineapple (for baked cherry pudding and apricot almond tart), boysenberries or raspberries (for apricot and pistachio risotto)

INGREDIENT INFORMATION

• Xanthan gum

Xanthan gum is a powder available from health food stores, and health food sections of larger supermarkets. It improves the quality of wheat free baking by enhancing the crumb structure. If xanthan gum is unavailable, guar gum or CMC (carboxymethyl cellulose) can be used.

• Fine rice flour

Fine rice flour can be purchased in the Asian section of the supermarket or from Asian grocers. Regular rice flour can be used, but it may result in a more textured final product.

• Potato flour

Potato flour is usually found in the health food section of supermarkets or in health food stores.

• Tapioca flour

Tapioca flour is usually found in the Asian section of supermarkets, or can be purchased from Asian grocers.

• Soy flour

Soy flour is usually found in the health food section of supermarkets or health food stores. If you have a soy intolerance, soy flour can be substituted with besan (chickpea) flour.

OTHER NOTES

Ingredients in *Irresistibles for the Irritable* are often indicated to specifically choose "gluten free". If this is not indicated, it is because the ingredient is naturally gluten free. Brand names of the specified gluten free ingredients have not been used, as manufacturers can change their recipe formulation. An insert will usually accompany *Irresistibles for the Irritable* with your purchase, indicating gluten free brands of ingredients used within the book. If you do not have the insert, or would like an up to date copy, it can be obtained from the website www.coeliac.com.au

There is no one gluten free grain or starch that is a perfect substitute for wheat in gluten free cooking. Recipes for cakes and biscuits may use a combination of more than one flour, to produce a much better quality product. Although it may seem more time consuming in the preparation than wheat based cooking, the improved final product is worth the extra effort.

All measurements in this cookbook are Australian standard measures. 1 cup = 250ml, 1 Tbsp = 20ml, 1 tsp = 5 ml. Residents of USA, Canada, UK and New Zealand will need to adjust recipes to their standard Tbsp = 15ml. Eggs used are 59g.